AF409519

A JOURNEY OF HEALTH

Routes and Advice from a Psychiatrist

Dr. Miguel Hernández

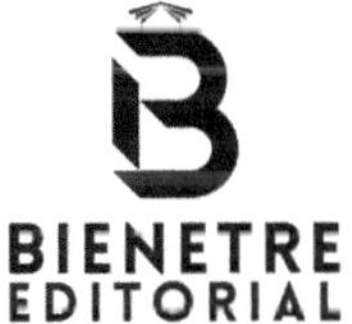

BIENETRE EDITORIAL

A JOURNEY OF HEALTH

Dr. Miguel Hernández

Published by Editorial Bien-etre.

Design and Page layout: Easwara Jiménez

Book cover design: Esteban Aquino

Illustrations: Elmer A. Hernández | Armani E. Hernández.

ISBN: 978-9945-647-23-5

Editing: Edited by Editorial Bien-etre.

Translation: Editorial Bien-etre.

First Edition 2023

Table of Contents

Acknowledgments

To my beloved Mother. Thank you for being everything in my existence. I love you.

To my sister, for your love and for being an important part of our lives.

To my Father, Ernesto Rafael Almánzar, my paternal cousins and brothers, especially Mateo Caba. To all my maternal family, especially to my dear uncles, aunts, and cousins. To my godmother, Lourdes Hernández.

To my dear wife Olga, thank you for your love, for being a wife, an exemplary mother, and an angel in my life.

To my beloved sons, Elmer and Armani, I love you with all my heart. Thank you for collaborating on this book with your childhood drawings.

To my pets, from Freud, Misunangu to Fuzzy.

To my childhood friends and my lifelong people from Ensanche Julia, UFE evening school and medical career in PUCMM. Especially to one of my Mentors, the outstanding psychiatrist of Santiago, Dr. José Joaquín Zouain, who passed away.

To the fraternities and sorors of the world, especially those of the pronaos of Santiago de los Caballeros, among them, Adalina García and Onésimo, to all those of the Manhattan chapter and the Brooklyn lodge, especially Jacqueline Disla and Aurelia García.

To my USA Army SFC friends, Santiago Cuellar, Shelly Eisert and her husband.

To colleagues and friends of the Dominican Medical Association of New York, Dominican Medical Center, especially Dr. Fernando Taveras, Virginia Taveras, Narcisa Taveras and Dr. Giovanny Núñez. To the primary and specialist physicians and health personnel of the community, Dominican Dental Medical Society, Somos and APHSI, especially Dr. Juan Tapia. To the medical and administrative leadership at NewYork–Presbyterian Hospital, Allen Hospital, Columbia University and Montefiore Mount Vernon, particularly Millie Onofrietti and Dr. Von Schorn. Special thanks to Dr. Casilda Balmaceda for providing me with information for one of the articles and Dr. Kelania Jiménez for being a collaborator on one of them. To my mentors and colleagues in the USA, Dr. Luisa González, Dr. Olusegun Bello, Dr. Henry Mcurtis, Dr. Evaristo Akarele, Dr. Melvin Gibert, Dr. Isaac Bampoe, Dr. Moisés Martínez, Dr. Ivelisse Capellán, Dr. Cristina Ovalles and Dr. Tresha Gibbs. To my colleagues in the Dominican Republic, Dr. Fernando López, Dr. Pedro Compres, Dr. Mirlan de Los Santos, Dr. Karin Mustafá, Dr. Ramón Estrella father and son, Dr. Fausto Valdez, Dr. Jesús Pastor Núñez Reyes and Dr. Sócrates Castillo. To the outstanding Dominican psychiatrist, Dr. César Mella, who was kind enough to write the foreword to this book.

To my brother and uncle Dr. José Contreras and his family; to the esteemed doctors, Dr. Roberto Morán and Dr. Robert Valenzuela.

To the lion brothers of all the jungles, especially Margarita Guerra, her husband, Dr. Aponte, Francia Mendoza and Manuel Núñez.

To Verbum Dei. Thank you Teresa, Raquel and all the people who serve spiritually.

My dear friends and brothers José N. García, Julio C. Báez, the late Santiago Vásquez and all the members of the trip to India and the Vedic astrology classes.

To the former leaders and directors of the Dominican American Round Table of the USA. To the representatives of the banks and financial institutions, Fulgence x Kabore, Howard Brachfeld, Ric Aberion, Yasandra Mercado, Yaniris Núñez, Elba Arias, Mercedes M. Mier, Dinangely Feliz, Yohanny Antonio and Rocío Adames.

To the dear brothers and sisters-in-law of all orientations, especially to the dear brothers of fraternity 387, José Beronio, his wife Laura, Hermes Mena and all the members of the lodge under dispensation Juan Pablo Duarte in the USA, especially Wylie Adames, Pedro Fraquer and Victor Escorbores.

To the people who helped me during the process of strengthening Miguel R. Hernández MD PC. To Aurelio Henríquez, Billy Francisco, Tony de la Rosa, Neris Jiménez, Ercilia García, writer and psychologist Ricardo Vacca, Dr.

Jorge Corniel, Dr. Héctor Reyes, Franklyn Morel and Dr. Pinkas I. Also, to all former employees and providers.

To the staff of Global Psychiatric Services PC, especially Nataly Grullón for her vital support to the company, as well as to all consultants and external companies for their services, CPA Lucy C., attorneys Antonio C. Martínez and A. García, HRC C. Goris, Nano printing and billers Roy R., Sharda S. and P. Cornielle.

To the dear members of the radio, television and photographic press. Especially to María Hiraldo and Nelson Encarnación, who gave me the opportunity to one day write for their newspaper Gaceta Hispana. To Zunilda Foundeur, Mayra La Paz, Pedro Morillo, Dr. Mejía Torres, Adalberto Domínguez, Nazario Brea, Federico Martínez (el Pacha), Dr. Eliecer Guzmán, David Rivas, Dra. Esmeldy Rosario, Ramón Darío Jiménez, César Romero, Yvonne Ramírez, Carolina Crespo, Italia Vignieri, Eddy Heredia, Nolagko Nolasco, Liany Ferreras, Kevin Martínez, Miguelina Rodríguez, Lina Beltre, Lewis Germán, Richie Hernández, Matibel, Ramón Aníbal Ramos, Roberto Gerónimo, Rafael Díaz, Frank Adolfo, Dr. Pedro Taveras, Miguel Estrella, José Alduey Sierra, José Samboy, Wilfredo Muñoz, Julio Colón Santana, Alex Hermoso, Manuel Sierra, Iván Morales, José Zabala, Francia Mendoza and Manuel Ruíz. To Keila González, director of Bienetre Editorial and María Trusa, director and CEO of Forme Medical Center.

To the community Leaders, dear Elida Almonte, Wilma Tamayo Abreu and writer Lourdes Batista.

To my friends in art, poetry and cinema, especially Anyeli Suárez, Monchi Herrera, Mariluz Acosta, Angie Regina, Billy Marte, Domingo Ramos and wife Dulce Ramos, Wilton Reinoso, Eduardo Luna, Danilo Arroyo, Eddy Jiménez, William Colmenares, Sugeiri Cristian, Susana Silfa, Yaneli Sosa, Génesis Tavárez, Ronald Sterling, Héctor Palacios, Antonio Rubio and Oirgo Papoutsas.

Elected officials, the Honorable Adriano Espaillat and Carmen de la Rosa.

To my chess friends from Santiago de los Caballeros and the Dominican Republic. Especially to the Vargas Brothers, Blas, Leo Estévez and Dr. Juan Luis Abreu. In the United States, Juan Villar and all the colleagues who every year make possible the Chess tournament that bears my name.

Because perhaps without knowing it, it was those micro and macro fragments of interaction with each one of you, that, in one way or another, made it possible for me to write all these articles that today are born as a book, which remains for the consideration of all of you and the rest of the world. Please forgive any unintentional omission of anyone important to the realization of this book.

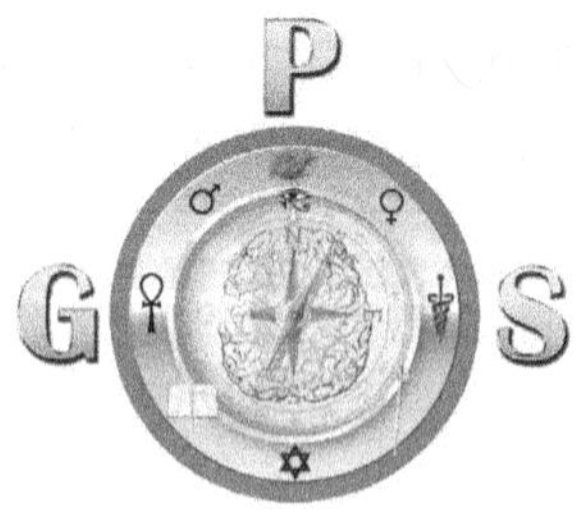

Foreword

The book you have in your hands results from the effort and dedication of a psychiatrist who lives and works in the United States.

Dr. Miguel Hernández graduated from the well-accredited Universidad Católica Madre y Maestra in Santiago de los Caballeros, Dominican Republic, where he also assisted a professor. Since then, he has not ceased studying, educating, disseminating, and ascending the difficult career and academic ladder in the United States based in prestigious institutions in New York.

For a psychiatrist with 40 years of practice, it is an honor and a distinction to be allowed to prologue this work, which is full of wisdom and of great utility for the reader of all levels.

First, what attracted my attention when I concluded reading this book? The author's power of communication makes the complex terms of our specialty easy to digest. In addition, the diversity of topics that put within popular reach ethical aspects of mental health and the concern for Hispanics living in the United States.

Various years ago, in a resort in the east of the Dominican Republic, I met Dr. Hernández. He told me he was working on a book and that he was inviting me to write the foreword; I was the president of the Latin American Psychiatric Association (APAL). I had forgotten him and, meanwhile, he was studying to receive the Licenses (Board) that would allow him to practice Psychiatry in the USA.

As the entrepreneur he is, Dr. Hernández has given lectures, conferences, and publications in the U.S. and abroad to complete an enviable curriculum vitae that has earned him high recognition from social institutions.

Dr. Hernández is the chairman of the board of directors of the Dominican Medical Association of New York and a member of the APA, the American Psychiatric Association.

This book has three parts that are easy to read:

I) MEDICAL ETHICS - THERE, HE ASKS AND ANSWERS HIMSELF:

Being a doctor? It means sacrifice, dedication, love for humanity and for the ill.

The doctor: his friends; the one who abuses substances; the success of the professional and its dangers, etc.

The doctor in front of COVID-19.- In which he narrates the suicide of the doctor, head of the emergency room of a renowned hospital in New York City.

Two issues deserve special reading: professional secrecy and the stigma that mental illness produces at a personal and family level.

II) MENTAL ILLNESSES

The author makes a didactic overview of depressions, post-traumatic stress, Mood Disorders (depressions), dementias, fibromyalgia, and others.

For each section, the author explains in plain language what they are, where they come from, how they are treated, and more:

He acknowledges his contributors and provides e-mail addresses of sources where the reader can expand on the topic.

The examples of his practice treating Hispanics and keeping their names secret are a guide drawn from the conditions and interaction with his patients.

III) SOCIAL PSYCHIATRY

Throughout these chapters, the reader will find clear and objective concepts of each topic.

I invite all readers in Latin America who wish to familiarize themselves with Mental Health from the perspective of an experienced psychiatrist who has positioned himself on the recognized Amazon platform, and I assure you that you will take A Journey of Health. I am convinced that his vision of life and the world will enrich you.

Dr. César Mella

Psychiatrist from the Dominican Republic

This book has been created to provide information on general aspects of mental health and medicine. The author, contributors, editors, and publishers do not intend to offer any legal, ethical, medical or mental health advice to be used as a treatment or substitute for treatment. Furthermore, it is not intended to establish a doctor-patient relationship with readers. Similarly, this book does not contain all the information available in the scientific literature on the topics discussed in it, so it cannot be used as a medical or mental health guide.

If you, a family member, or friend is ill and needs medical or psychiatric treatment, please consult your primary care physician, mental health provider or go to the nearest emergency room.

The author, contributors, editors, and publishers shall not incur any legal liability or be held responsible if any damages of any kind occur directly or indirectly from the use of the information contained in this book.

The author has no conflict of interest with corporations, firms, or companies in the pharmaceutical, laboratory, medical, mental health or other health services industries. Nothing to declare.

By continuing to read beyond this page, you confirm your agreement to this disclaimer.

CHAPTER I:

Medical Doctors and Medicine

The Practice of Being a Doctor
Vocation or Business?

We live in a society bombarded with information and loaded with great subjectivity, which is supported by pseudo-truths. As a result, we find that the behavior of many professional and non-professional people is changing unfavorably. Over time, the roots of human collective knowledge grow in inappropriate directions. These inappropriate directions lead to negative actions, which are then reinforced and rewarded by the media. Actions and influence at all social levels often cannot be stopped, altered, or destroyed by any ideology, including political, legal, moral, philosophical, or religious beliefs.

Many well-known books use imagination to present reality as a lady dressed in historical truth and become bestsellers with millions of copies sold. On the other hand, politicians often win elections by making false promises in their campaigns. These can range from using old, heavily edited photos on posters to promising great projects and changes that are rarely completed. Likewise, great powers often maintain their success by taking advantage of poor countries and treating them as modern colonies. At the same time, they are praised by the international press for their diplomatic skills and commitment to world peace.

Many countries are struggling with corruption, violence, and poverty, yet we often give children cell phones and computers without teaching them basic social etiquette such as saying "good morning," controlling their language, offering a seat on public transportation, and asking permission to pass between people. In a world where wrongdoers are often celebrated and money is more important than dignity, the best values are disappearing, even in traditionally respected professions like medicine.

Dr. Murad Malik Mustafá (not his real name) was born in a Middle Eastern country and has been working in the United States for over 20 years. He has a specialized private practice and is a full time attending at a prestigious metropolitan area hospital in Bronx, New York. A few years ago, while visiting his clinic with a family member, I asked him for advice on which subspecialty to choose in my career. I was finishing my specialty in Psychiatry at the time. His response was:

"Medicine here in the United States is not like in our countries, where the physician is valued as a God, treated and trusted as if he were family. In most cases, the doctor offers a high-quality service because he sees the patient as a lawsuit threat and not as a human being full of feelings and needs. I think you should choose the best paid, regardless of whether you like it or not."

Dr. Murad Malik Mustafa's opinion reflects the way of conceiving today's majority of physicians in many countries of the world. It is alarming that this materialistic world is slowly causing us to lose touch with our purest and most romantic selves, which once motivated us to pursue careers in medicine to help others. As a result, we end up with empty doctors who are only in it for the money, rather than seeing the profession as a way to transcend spiritually and make a true difference in the world as it was once intended.

Medicine as a pure business and not as a vocation represents one of the many dangers that threaten the harmony of humanity. Fortunately, there are many who believe that it is still possible to turn things around and that one day the profession of Hippocrates, Galen, and Paracelsus can return to being a business of sacrifice, humility, and love for others.

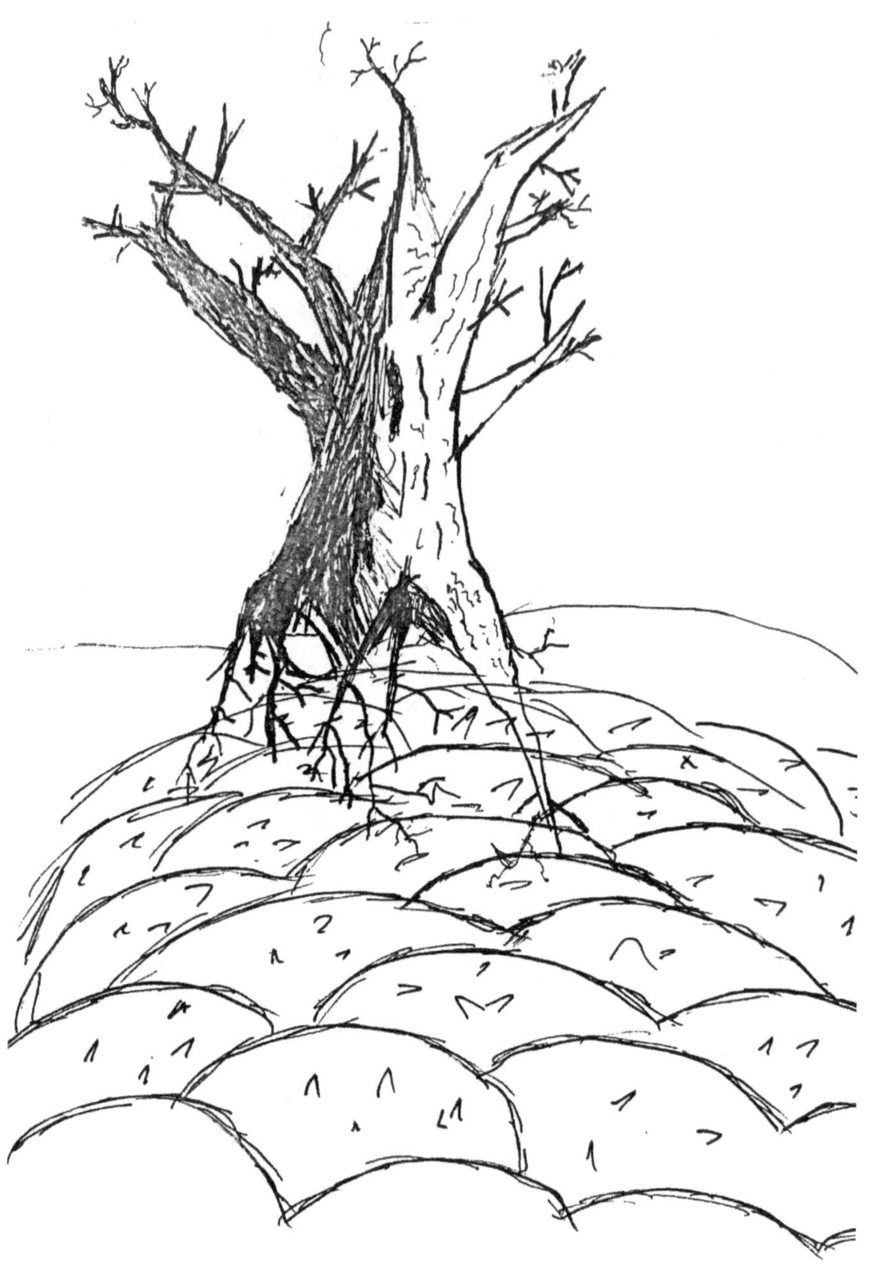

Doctors and their Friends
Professional Duty vs. Fraternal Risk

There may be times when a physician's friendships could be jeopardized if the boundaries between friendship and medical practice are not clearly defined.

It is natural to want to have a friend to call on for advice on where to go, what to take, or what to do in case of illness. It can be extremely helpful to have someone to confide in and receive wise advice from. Imagine the convenience of being able to consult with your doctor friend on the street, while on vacation, on public transportation, or at home during a party. It can bring peace of mind to be able to call your doctor friend on the phone to solve a problem or seek ideas on how to solve it, almost 24 hours a day, all year long.

At first glance, it seems fortunate to have a close family doctor or trusted friend, perhaps someone you've known since childhood, and we might think: "That's what friends are for, right?". However, our perspective may change when we consider the challenges and negative consequences for a physician's job position that can come with having to be flexible and accommodate friends or acquaintances in hospital or clinic settings, who do not understand the legal and ethical differences between common practices in their countries and those in the United States.

It is human nature to have a high level of trust in authority figures like doctors, and this is not just a cultural trait that immigrants carry with them. However, regardless of culture, when trust becomes harmful, even unintentionally, we must stop and be more cautious to avoid damaging a good relationship.

For example, there are many people who become angry and doubt the genuineness of a friendship when a doctor is unable to give them a prescription, diagnostic test, medical certificate, get them an early appointment at a colleague's clinic, see them without an appointment, or see them for free. Many may believe that the doctor lacks compassion or dedication to their profession if they refuse to fulfill all requests made in the name of "friendship", without considering the reality that a responsible physician has a moral and professional duty to uphold.

Elena Álvarez (not her real name), a U.S.-born geriatric internist of Dominican descent practicing in Houston, Texas, told me that she has seen this type of behavior more frequently among Hispanic friends and patients. She also emphasized the importance of being vigilant in these situations and of setting limits with friends who ask for favors that would go beyond what she can provide without harming herself.

There is another, more subtle risk in physician friendships

(note that we are not referring to the physician-patient relationship) that both the physician and the friend may not be aware of. This risk occurs when more information is shared in a friendship than would be shared in a normal relationship, simply because the friend is a physician. The information is often shared with the disclaimer "I say this to you because you are a physician, but don't tell anyone else."

We must be responsible for determining whether secrets are shared with us because we are considered friends or because we are physicians. As my colleague said, we must immediately set limits and clearly express how harmful it can be to distort friendship by sharing information, often pseudo-voluntarily, based on professional status.

Physicians, like other professionals, have the right to enjoy their friendships and have friends enjoy their company, just as they did before obtaining their university degree. They can do so without jeopardizing their friendships, without forgetting their professional duty, and without sacrificing mutual respect that comes from pure love.

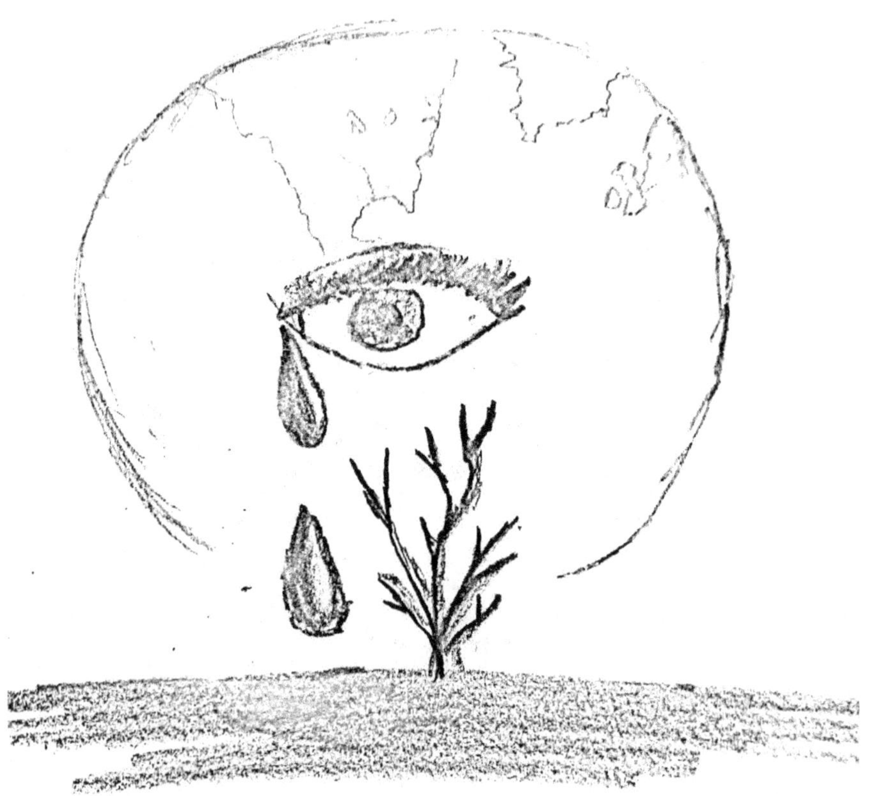

Doctors and Professional Success
Sacrifice vs. Wellness

Every professional remembers the sacrifices made during their career journey. Most of us understand how challenging it is to succeed in a competitive field and remain relevant. For physicians and other professionals, the drive to succeed often comes from a desire for self-improvement and the ambition to achieve well-being in all aspects of life.

Success brings many benefits. These include material benefits like the ability to afford a nice home or car and take vacations. They also include social benefits like attaining high social status and engaging in philanthropic activities. Finally, they include future security benefits like the ability to retire early and provide education for children.

Medical salaries can range from $130,000 to $350,000 per year. However, physicians are often among the most demanding professionals, working more than 60 hours a week and dedicating much of their personal time to advanced studies, courses, conferences, and certification updates. As a result, well-being may be limited to economic and material benefits, while other important aspects of life, like relationships with family and friends, are neglected.

This sacrifice can lead to neglect of children, spouses, and other loved ones, potentially resulting in divorce, poorly educated children, drug use, loneliness, feelings of guilt, and ultimately, depression. Additionally, some individuals may neglect their own physical and mental health and fail to prioritize preventative care or seek timely treatment, leading to deterioration of their health. Some may also abandon their spiritual practices and cease cultivating their philosophical and religious beliefs.

The story of Miguel López (not his real name), a Dominican physician practicing in a Massachusetts hospital, exemplifies the challenges discussed. He works 12-hour shifts, sometimes more, at least 4 times a month, in addition to his regular 9-hour schedule. He worries that this demanding schedule may cause marital conflicts, and has had to stop attending church regularly on Saturdays.

In conclusion, we must be mindful as we pursue success, as the pursuit itself can distract us from our true purpose in life and cause us to lose sight of what truly matters to us. As the popular Dominican saying goes, "more salt than goat" (*más la sal que el chivo*).

Doctors and Substance Abuse

Sober Truths that Intoxicate

In the United States, it is estimated that approximately 9-14% of the population suffers from a substance use disorder. Physicians are affected in the same proportion as the general population, however, there are significant differences in this particular group that are important to mention and analyze.

In physicians, substance use can begin during their student days, with drugs similar to those used by the general population, such as alcohol, tobacco, or marijuana. It can then continue during residency and into medical practice. In these stages, the misuse of opium-derived drugs and benzodiazepines in the form of self-prescription is five times more frequent. Reasons for use among physicians are varied, including recreation, improved job performance, and self-medication for anxiety, stress, and depression.

In both physicians and anyone who abuses these substances, the gradual deterioration manifests in areas such as physical and emotional health, finances, family, and work performance. Eventually, abuse turns into dependence and social obligations become increasingly difficult to fulfill. The substance is no longer used to feel good, but to avoid feeling bad.

Even when trapped by dependence, many physicians, believing themselves to be independent and hiding behind their level of knowledge, refuse to accept the reality of their condition. Fearing negative consequences for their reputation, they remain silent and delay seeking professional help.

Other factors that hinder early identification and treatment in physicians with substance use disorder include professional pride, the threat of losing the respect of society, risk of financial loss, and the difficulty of reversing roles to become a patient while being a physician.

It is important for everyone to be aware of the signs of substance abuse or dependence in themselves, their family members, friends, or patients, whether they are physicians or not. We should educate ourselves and avoid thinking like many Latinos who say "I am not an alcoholic because I only drink on weekends" or "Sometimes I take a 'pass' when I am out having fun."

Despite the obstacles to accepting the condition, seeking help, and early identification, there is good news: substance abuse treatment has better outcomes in physicians than in the general population. Treatment success rates are over 80%, regardless of the physician's specialty or the type of substance used.

Additionally, for Hispanic physicians, the risk of substance use and abuse, including alcohol, is much higher during holidays such as Christmas, and the risk of relapse in abstinent patients is also increased. We urge colleagues and the general population to be aware of this risk and to seek alternative ways of coping during these celebrations.

In conclusion, physicians should be aware of their habits and strive to maintain abstinence as much as possible. If they are already trapped in a substance use disorder, they should be honest with themselves and immediately seek help from family or friends, and seek professional assistance.

Medicine and Cultural Sensitivity
Hand in Hand Make a Big Difference

Cultural sensitivity plays a crucial role in the diagnostic and therapeutic process of patients, especially in a multicultural country like the United States. Inadequate cultural sensitivity can lead to patients dropping out of treatment, not following through with therapy, or experiencing negative consequences from medical decisions.

Even though interpreters are available in most US healthcare facilities, difficulties can still arise from a lack of knowledge of the patient's cultural context. This is particularly likely when the therapist does not belong to the same ethnic group as the patient or has not received sufficient cultural sensitivity training. For example, in a psychiatric evaluation, an interpreter's translation of a symptom or thought could lead to an involuntary hospital admission or discharge if the evaluator is unfamiliar with the patient's cultural background.

Furthermore, the therapeutic alliance can be weakened when the physician does not understand that some patients prefer home remedies, or seek advice from healers or spiritual guides, rather than following the physician's recommendations. Moreover, certain cultures may believe that illnesses are caused by supernatural forces.

There are numerous cultural syndromes in medicine, which may have different names depending on the cultural group. For instance, Caribbean Latinos may experience "nervous breakdown" which is characterized by uncontrollable screaming, shortness of breath, feeling of being out of control, tremors, dizziness and so on, which may happen when the individual face great stressors.

Similarly, in West Africa we can find "exhausted or tired brain", which occurs in highly studious young people and is characterized by difficulty concentrating, loss of memory and thinking. Some people report it as their brain being fatigued.

Another example is Koro, which is prevalent in South and East Asia, is an intense episode of anxiety and worry that the penis, vagina, or nipples could shrink in size until they disappear inside the body and cause death. We could continue mentioning many others such as "nervios", "mal de ojo", "locura", "susto", "zar", "piblokto", among others, that we can find in different regions of the world.

In conclusion, understanding and cultural sensitivity are essential for medical practice. It is challenging to understand the values, meanings, and different behaviors "normal" to certain ethnic groups, but it is without doubt that when medicine is paired with cultural sensitivity, the therapeutic path is illuminated with benefits for both the physician and the patient.

Moral Injury in Health Professionals during the COVID-19 Pandemic

Contagious Mental Trauma of a Global Disaster

At the end of April 2021, the SARS-2 coronavirus, responsible for COVID-19, had affected over three million individuals and caused 233,000 deaths worldwide. The United States had the highest numbers, with over one million confirmed cases and 73,000 deaths (according to data from John Hopkins University's CSSE).

On March 11th, 2020, the World Health Organization declared the outbreak a pandemic, citing its ability to meet the combination of elements that defines a disaster, as defined by Enrico Quarantelli. However, it breaks with the emotional sequencing of disaster victims as described by Farberow and Gordon in 1981, due to its viral pandemic nature (John D. Weaver, Disasters: mental health interventions, p. 7, 31).

Government authorities, the press, and the general public have mainly focused on increasing the availability of personal protective equipment, handwashing, social distancing and other infection prevention measures for healthcare personnel. While this is commendable, there has been a lack of attention to the mental health of healthcare workers, with no immediate interventions or long-term plans in place for sustainable treatment.

This omission may lead to an increase in the risk of anxiety disorders, depression, post-traumatic stress disorder, and suicide, particularly among front-line healthcare workers who are involved in direct treatment of COVID-19 patients, such as nurses and female staff (as per reference to the studies of JianboLai, JAMA Netw Open. 2020; Moral Injury: EldoFrezza Md Tex Med 2019).

Since the outbreak of the pandemic, the media has highlighted the struggles faced by essential front-line workers, particularly nurses and doctors. Images and videos shared on social media and television depicted these individuals wearing protective masks, often visibly exhausted and emotional, reflecting the uncertainty, helplessness, and despair they were experiencing.

In New York, the epicenter of the pandemic, the number of patients requiring care has significantly outstripped the availability of healthcare workers. Additionally, paramedics, nurses, and doctors are working hours that are beyond what is typical in the U.S. healthcare system. It is imperative that efforts are made to protect the working hours of doctors in medical residencies under the Libby Zion law, despite the extreme circumstances of the crisis.

A video of Dr. Jessica Gold[1] discussing moral injury, which caught our attention, highlights the impact of the situation.

---

[1] Assistant Professor at Washington University In St. Louis, Missouri. She speaks via Medpage.com

She shared a message from her friend Dr. Craig Spencer, who works in the emergency room of a New York hospital. The message describes the pain, loneliness and death that the physician and his colleagues are facing. Constant alarms alerting them to another patient having a cardiac arrest, and the hard choices of which patient to treat first to avoid death, are just some examples he shared.

This illustrates the traumatic and devastating experience healthcare workers are facing, who are trained to save lives, it is not only an issue in the US but also a global problem, healthcare workers in countries like China, Spain, Italy, Iran, Ecuador, and the Dominican Republic are also facing this humanitarian crisis.

On April 26 of this year, Dr. Lorna Breen[2] took her own life, a tragic reminder of the emotional stress faced by healthcare workers, which is compounded by the scale of the crisis that has affected the entire globe. This was followed two days later, in Queens County, New York, where a paramedic also took his own life, it demonstrates the gravity of the emotional burden that healthcare workers have been coping with during the pandemic.

Moral injury refers to the emotional and psychological harm caused by actions or events that fundamentally contradict an individual's moral beliefs and expectations. This can occur when a person is forced to participate in, or witness, behaviors

---

[2] She was in charge of the emergency department of the Allen Pavilion of the Presbyterian Hospital in New York.

that violate their ethical values. Examples include soldiers being required to kill enemies in war, or healthcare workers being unable to save patients due to a lack of resources. The resulting guilt, shame, and betrayal can lead to significant psychological stress and changes in behavior. The harm is reflected in the aftermath that follows exposure to the events, which is often experienced with a level of psychological stress and behavioral change. This type of injury is often seen in individuals who are in situations where they must act or witness behaviors that are against their moral and ethical values[3].

Moral injury should not be confused with burnout, as the latter suggests that the problem lies with the sufferer rather than the system, which skews the perspective of the source of the problem and thus diverts the focus of the solution (Wendy Dean, MD Fed Pract. 2019; 36(9): 400-402). To properly measure and understand moral injury, there are diagnostic tools available, such as the 20-item Moral Injury Questionnaire (MIQ, 18) and the 9-item Moral Injury Events Scale (MIES, 20).

The Mount Sinai Health System in New York City has been heroically supporting its health care staff. The support group found three core priorities for maintaining the well-being of its staff during the pandemic: meeting basic daily needs, increasing communication of up-to-date, reliable, and reassuring messages, and developing robust psychological and mental health support options (Jonathan Ripp, Acad Med. 2020).

---

[3] www.ptsd.va.gov, www.menteforense.com

Treatment for moral injury in healthcare workers can be challenging, as patients may feel ashamed or fearful of judgment from mental health providers. However, research has shown that therapies such as prolonged exposure therapy and cognitive processing therapy, which are also used for post-traumatic stress disorder, can be effective for patients with moral injury as well (Sonya B. Norman, PhD).

The American Medical Association (AMA) has provided the following recommendations to physicians to help combat stress during the pandemic:

- Prioritizing basic needs such as nourishment, hydration, safety, and adequate sleep.

- Monitoring work hours and taking breaks as necessary, with the healthcare system ensuring that this happens.

- Making mental health resources available and easily accessible.

- Showing compassion and empathy from leaders towards physicians' experiences on the frontline of the crisis and addressing their concerns and fears.

- Effectively distributing the workload and fostering a culture of wellness within the workplace by providing moral support to one another.

In order for healthcare professionals to effectively manage the impacts of the COVID-19 pandemic, it is important for them to understand the concept of moral injury, its potential to cause trauma and its negative impact on mental health. This includes understanding the specific ways that moral injury can occur within their work environment. With this knowledge, they will be better equipped to identify and address moral injury in themselves and their colleagues, to prevent it or seek help as needed.

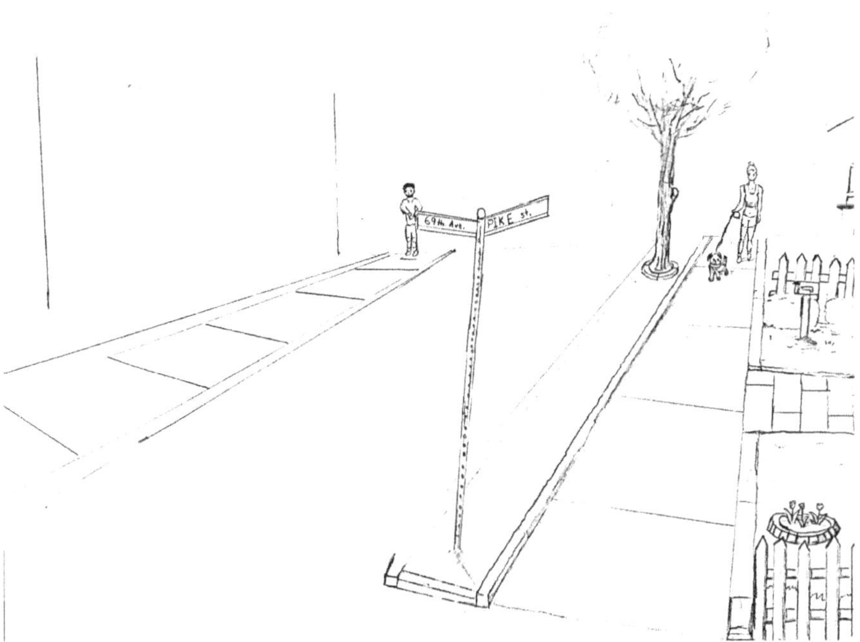

CHAPTER II:

Psychiatric Illnesses

Psychiatric Emergencies
Situations of Imminent Risk of Death

Psychiatric emergencies may be commonly associated with high-profile incidents portrayed by media, such as an individual with a mental illness threatening to commit suicide from a tall structure, and the efforts of authorities and mental health professionals to intervene. However, it's important to note that psychiatric emergencies are not solely caused by mental illness and can occur frequently in different forms. These emergencies require action without delay to save the life of the patient or others and avoid other serious consequences (Dtsch Arztebl Int., 2011).

In the United States, there were an estimated 4.3 million psychiatry-related emergency department visits in the year 2000. This translates to an annual rate of 21 visits per 1,000 adults (Acad Emerg Med. 2004). This trend has been observed in other areas, specifically in New York where the number of psychiatric emergency department visits saw a significant increase between 1976 and 1988, with an estimated 135,000 emergency evaluations being performed annually (Dawes SS University of Albany, 1995).

Depending on the patient's symptoms, it may be necessary to conduct a medical and neurological examination, as well as blood and urine tests, to rule out or confirm the presence of any underlying medical or substance-related causes. In cases where the diagnosis is not clear, additional diagnostic tools such as computed tomography, magnetic resonance imaging, and other laboratory studies may be used.

The intervention and treatment of psychiatric emergencies is a complex process. If verbal persuasion, environmental modifications, behavioral therapy, and pharmacological restraints are ineffective, mechanical restraint may be used as a last resort to control high-risk behaviors that threaten the safety of the patient, other patients, or healthcare professionals. This may be necessary for patients experiencing agitation, confusion, delirium, suicidal or homicidal ideation, or altered consciousness.

Medical and psychiatric staff must be able to quickly and confidently determine when acute treatment and involuntary commitment is necessary, and not be swayed by requests for discharge against medical advice from patients, friends, or family members.

The choice of pharmacological treatment and administration route will depend on the patient's specific symptoms, history, and diagnosis. Commonly used medications include antipsychotics such as haloperidol, chlorpromazine, ziprasidone, aripiprazole, olanzapine, asenapine, and benzodiazepines such as lorazepam, diazepam, clozapine, and chlordiazepoxide. These drugs may be used alone or in combination as appropriate. The most common route of administration is intramuscular injection, but intravenous and oral routes may also be used in certain scenarios.

If you or someone you know is experiencing a psychiatric emergency, please seek help from the following options: contacting your physician or an on-call mental health professional, calling 911, 1-800-Lifenet or 1-800-Ayudese, or bringing the affected person to the nearest medical or psychiatric emergency room, considering the need for police or security presence based on the severity of the situation.

For information about mental illness: 1-866-615-NIMH (6464) (the call Is free for those living in the United States).

E-mail: nimhinfo@nih.gov

Web site: http://www.nimh.nih.gov

DR. MIGUEL HERNÁNDEZ

The Social Stigma of Mental Illnesses

Indelible Scars of Ignorance

According to the U.S. National Institute of Mental Health (NIMH), approximately 26.2% of the U.S. population aged 18 and older, or nearly 58 million people, are affected by a diagnosable mental disorder. This represents one in four adults. While mental illness is prevalent globally, the societal stigma associated with it continues to have a negative impact on those who are affected.

Individuals with mental illnesses not only experience the direct effects of their illness, but also the challenges of societal ignorance and discrimination. This bias often exacerbates the difficulties they face in terms of social and occupational integration. Negative societal attitudes can create additional barriers that increase the risk of isolation and marginalization (Muñoz, 2009).

The lack of public education and understanding about mental illnesses, their causes, and treatment contribute to discrimination against those with mental disorders. People may avoid seeking help for fear of being labeled as mentally ill, which can lead to loss of employment or future job opportunities, exclusion from leadership roles in society, rejection by friends and family, and other negative consequences.

Many public figures, such as politicians, actors, television personalities, and athletes, freely and sometimes proudly announce when they or someone in their family has been diagnosed with conditions like cancer, diabetes, or HIV. However, relatively few publicly acknowledge conditions such as bipolar disorder, drug addiction, schizophrenia, anorexia nervosa, and others. This disparity is likely due to the misconceptions and social stigmas surrounding mental illness.

It is important to keep in mind the following points to help break these stigmas:

- Mental disorders, similar to what are referred to as "organic" diseases (e.g., diabetes, high blood pressure or asthma) are caused by both genetic and environmental factors and those who suffer from them are not at fault, nor do they want to or deserve to suffer from them.

- In the same way, as we do not view someone suffering from peptic ulcer or kidney disease as less important or capable, we should not view those with mental illnesses in that way.

- We should avoid derogatory terms such as "crazy," "retarded," or "idiot" when referring to those with mental illness and avoid placing blame on them for their symptoms. This is like not blaming a child for having stomach pain due to gastritis, a person with migraines for having a headache, or a person with cancer for losing weight. Likewise, we should not judge or belittle an individual who experiences sadness or irritability due to depression.

- The media also plays a significant role in perpetuating these stigmas and should be more responsible in their portrayal of those with mental illness, not depicting them as violent, dangerous, or criminal individuals.

In conclusion, it is important for us all to educate ourselves about mental illnesses, be more empathetic, and less judgmental of those who suffer from them. By doing so, we can work towards building a more fair and just society that is less discriminatory towards those with mental illnesses.

For information about bipolar and other mental illnesses: 1-866-615-NIMH (6464) (toll-free for those living in the United States). E-mail: nimhinfo@nih.gov / Website: http://www.nimh.nih.gov.

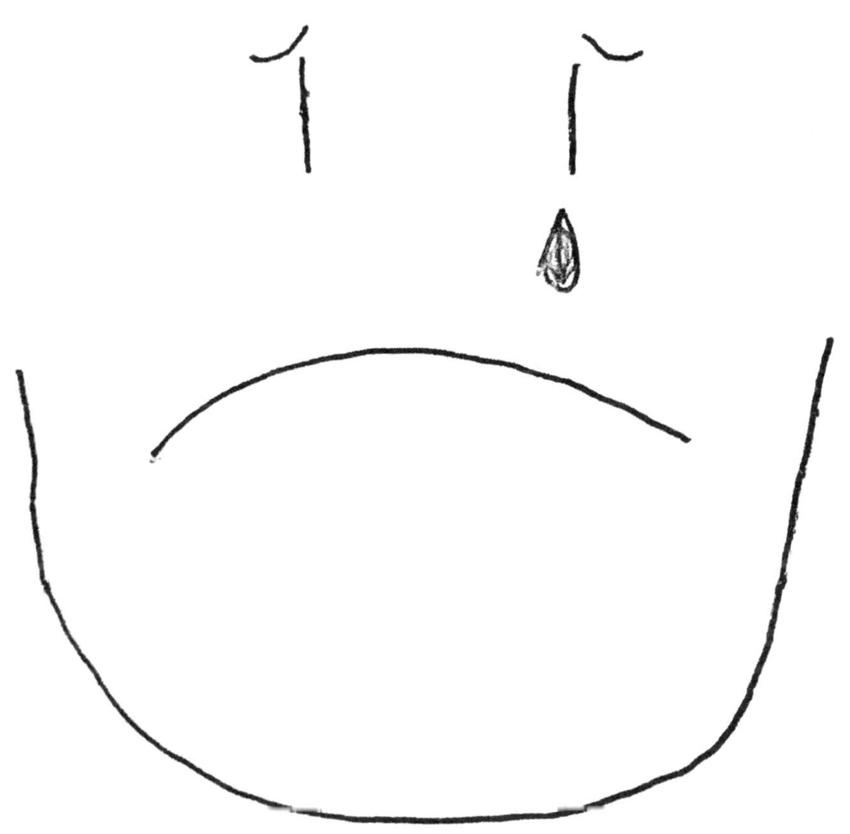

Mental Illness and Family

Knowledge vs. Ignorance

Every day, a large number of people around the world are affected by mental illness. The conditions are diverse: from children with attention deficit hyperactivity disorder, adolescents struggling with addiction, to elderly individuals with Alzheimer's disease.

Often, it is the family members of those with mental illness who suffer just as much, if not more, than the individuals affected. They are responsible for maintaining a stable and unconditionally supportive family environment that serves as a barrier against relapse and the progression of behavioral disorders. They may also be responsible for overseeing day-to-day activities such as personal hygiene, education, nutrition, finances, and even recreation for the family member with mental health challenges.

So far, this would be the same as if there were someone in the family suffering from an organic disease, such as diabetes, terminal cancer, multiple sclerosis, and myasthenia gravis. However, with mental illnesses, there is an additional challenge: the negative factor of the social stigma that comes with having a family member who is mistakenly labeled as "crazy" or "mad."

Furthermore, we know that in many cases, mental illnesses such as schizophrenia, bipolar disorder, alcohol abuse, and illicit drug abuse can impair judgment and decision-making abilities. This can lead to a denial of the illness and a rejection of treatment and/or help from family members.

Faced with the reality of dealing with the shame and frustration of what, to them, is inexplicable, feelings of guilt, hopelessness, and helplessness are born. As a result, they tend to cling to popular beliefs full of superstition and ignorance. Despite advances in science and educational propaganda about the biological and environmental etiology of mental illness, in Hispanic families, it is still very common to believe that mental diseases are a punishment from God, the result of witchcraft, or simply a behavioral predisposition learned in the streets or copied from a friend.

Doris Santos (not her real name) is a 32-year-old Hispanic woman born in the Dominican Republic who currently lives in the Bronx and works for a prestigious hotel chain in New York. She constantly accused her 8-year-old son of being lazy, like his father's family, because he had difficulty getting up early and going to school. She says she felt guilty and very bad when months later her child was diagnosed with depression.

Both Doris and we are convinced that no mother would accuse her child of having a fever or coughing in the middle of the night when they have the onset of bronchitis; however, Doris's son was being accused of laziness through no fault of his own for his inadequate brain functioning. One of the ways the brain manifests when it is sick with depression is through behavioral changes, just as the lung would with fever and cough if it were afflicted with bronchitis or pneumonia.

The case of Doris Santos demonstrates the lack of education that exists among family members of the mentally ill and the general population. Fortunately, organizations such as the National Alliance for the Mentally Ill (NAMI) provide nationwide education and support for the mentally ill and their families.

We believe that we are all responsible for educating society about the reality of mental illness to help eradicate the stigma, ignorance, and unfair discrimination that still exist. This would bring relief and peace of mind, not only to the sick, but also to their closest protectors: their families.

Personality Disorders

A Rainbow of Actions in Each Individual

A large part of the population is unaware of personality disorders, especially those outside the field of medicine. Furthermore, many do not even imagine that there is a psychiatric diagnosis referred to as "personality disorder." Since these deviant personality patterns lead individuals to a significant degree of stress and unhappiness, and because of their clinical relationship with other mental illnesses, it is appropriate to examine this topic. In doing so, we will extract the necessary information to understand the various shades of human personality.

The Diagnostic and Statistical Manual of Psychiatry (DSM-IV-TR) defines personality disorders as patterns of internal experience and behavior that deviate significantly from an individual's cultural expectations. These patterns are manifested in two or more of the following areas: cognitive (the way of perceiving and interpreting people, events, and oneself), affective, interpersonal relationships, and impulse control. Additionally, the manual states that these characteristics cause social dysfunction for the individual in an important area of their life. The behavior patterns are stable, long-lasting, and typically appear in adolescence or early adulthood.

The types of personality disorders have been classified into clusters A, B, and C based on their most prominent characteristics. Group A includes those personality types characterized by being almost always suspicious without reason, lacking trust in others, holding grudges, perceiving an attack in any comment, perceiving infidelities in their relationships without proof, etc. In this group, we have paranoid, schizotypal, and schizoid personality disorders.

In the same manner, group B includes individuals with patterns characterized by little respect for the rights of others, violation of the law and social norms, instability in interpersonal relationships, self-image, affection management, and impulse control, desire for attention, need for admiration, sense of grandeur and importance. As examples, we have antisocial personality disorders, also known as sociopaths, borderline personality disorders, narcissistic personality disorders, and histrionic personality disorders.

Cluster C includes individuals with patterns of social inhibition, hypersensitivity to negative evaluations, submissive characteristics, fear of separation from people, excessive need for others, and exaggerated preoccupation with order and perfection. Here we have dependent, obsessive-compulsive, and avoidant personality disorders.

Finally, it is important to reiterate that we are dealing with a true personality disorder when these patterns cause significant dysfunction in the individual, becoming rigid and prominent. Moreover, it's important to understand that we all have a little of each of the patterns described above. For this reason, some authors refer to these as personality styles in individuals without any personality disorder. Additionally, it should not be confused with dissociative identity disorders, traditionally known as multiple personality disorders.

Moreover, personality disorders are often "egosyntonic," meaning individuals are rarely aware that they have a disorder and therefore hardly ever seek professional help. We hope to delve more deeply into each type of disorder at a later occasion. We are sure that by then, we will be able to identify with some type of disorder and see it in a neighbor, a boss, a parent, a celebrity, a child, a spouse, or a friend.

Depression

The Sad Mask Behind Suicide

Mood or affective disorders, such as depression, continue to be a significant public health problem. According to the National Institute of Mental Health (NIMH), 9.5% of the population in the USA, or approximately 18.8 million adults, suffers from depression. This represents a high cost in both economic and human suffering. Alarmingly, 15 out of every 100 people with severe depression die by suicide. It is important to understand this issue and learn more about the sad reality of voluntary death.

Depression affects more women, individuals who are single or divorced, and occurs more frequently between the ages of 20 and 30, although it can also appear during childhood. Unfortunately, few seek help, and many are unaware that depression is treatable.

Depression is a brain disease that affects behavior. It is not a passing sadness during a difficult situation or bereavement, nor is it a voluntary choice or a characteristic of individuals. It is also not a sign of weakness or laziness, or a result of a spell or divine punishment.

Biological, genetic, and psychosocial factors play an important role in the origin of depression. Biological factors include the role of biogenic amines such as serotonin, epinephrine, and dopamine, as well as alterations in endocrine and neuroimmune regulation. Studies in twins and adopted children have also found evidence of a genetic predisposition to depression. Additionally, losing a parent before the age of 11 and losing a spouse are significant psychosocial stressors that can contribute to depression.

There are several types of affective disorders that manifest as depression. To be diagnosed with major or unipolar depression, an individual must experience five or more of the following symptoms for a minimum of two weeks, without having had a manic or hypomanic episode, and without the symptoms being caused by substance use: a sad or empty mood, thoughts of hopelessness, pessimism, guilt or helplessness, loss of interest or pleasure, low energy or fatigue, difficulty concentrating, changes in sleep patterns, changes in appetite, thoughts of suicide or death, restlessness, irritability, and physical symptoms.

Treatment for depression may include medication and/or psychotherapy, with a combination of both being more effective than a single intervention. It is important to note that antidepressant medication does not cause dependence, contrary to popular belief.

Just as with the use of illicit drugs and alcohol, there are certain natural remedies that can interact with and negatively affect the treatment of depression. One example is the use of serotonin reuptake inhibitors (such as fluoxetine, sertraline, or paroxetine) in combination with St. John's Wort tea, which is a commonly used natural remedy for improving symptoms of depression. Therefore, it is important to inform your doctor about any substances or medications you are taking before starting treatment for depression.

It's also worth noting that medications for depression can cause a variety of temporary side effects, though these are usually mild. Antidepressants typically take one to two weeks to fully take effect, and it is recommended that treatment with medication and/or psychotherapy be continued for a minimum of six months to one and a half years in order to reduce the risk of relapse.

In addition to medication and therapy, there are also self-help measures that can be helpful in managing depression. Some examples include setting realistic goals, talking to someone, engaging in light exercise, participating in recreational activities, postponing important decisions, cultivating positive thought patterns, and accepting help from others.

Postpartum Depression

Anguished Birth of Hormonal Vulnerability

Postpartum depression is a serious mental illness that involves the brain. It is estimated that around 7 to 13% of women in the postpartum period are affected by this mental disorder (NIMH). However, it is believed that this figure is higher, since like many other mental illnesses, perinatal depression is often not recognized and treated in time. We consider it of utmost importance to educate the population about this overwhelming condition for vulnerable mothers and families.

Postpartum depression is a serious mental illness that goes beyond feeling nostalgic or unmotivated. It is also referred to as postnatal depression, maternal depression, or perinatal depression. It should not be confused with "baby blues," a milder and temporary form of depression that affects approximately 70 to 80% of first-time mothers and is characterized by sadness, sleep problems, difficulty concentrating, worry, and emotional changes. Baby blues typically occurs between the fourth and fifth day after giving birth and resolves within 14 days after delivery. Postpartum depression can also affect men, although to a lesser extent, particularly in the case of first-time fathers.

Postpartum depression can affect any woman, regardless of her age, race, culture, or education. It affects mothers of healthy or sick babies equally, whether they breastfeed or not, are married or single, and experienced problems or not during pregnancy.

There are risk factors for developing postpartum depression, including a history of depression or bipolar disorder, alcohol or drug use or abuse, financial or relationship problems, a family history of affective disorders, little social support, being a single mother, low self-esteem, a previous episode of postpartum depression, an unwanted pregnancy, not breastfeeding the baby, low socioeconomic status, having a baby with a difficult temperament, smoking cigarettes, decreased levels of oxytocin, among others. It's important to note that some women may have multiple risk factors and still not develop postpartum depression, while others may not have any risk factors and still experience it.

The symptoms of postpartum depression can appear either right after childbirth or at any point during the first year after giving birth. Common symptoms include feelings of sadness, anxiety or excessive worrying, irritability or a bad mood, difficulty sleeping even when tired or sleeping too much, loss of interest in self-care, little or increased appetite, frequent crying for no apparent reason, exaggerated or minimal concern for the baby, and loss of pleasure or interest in things that were once enjoyed.

It's worth noting that a small percentage of women suffer from a more severe form of postpartum depression known as postpartum psychosis, which is characterized by extreme confusion, insomnia, loss of appetite, paranoia, visual and auditory hallucinations (seeing or hearing things that others cannot), thoughts of death or suicidal ideation, and plans to harm or kill the baby.

Postpartum psychosis is a psychiatric emergency and requires immediate medical intervention.

The evaluation and treatment of postpartum depression require a comprehensive medical evaluation, including blood and urine tests to rule out "organic or physiological" causes, psychotherapy, support groups, and psychotropic medication such as antidepressants.

It is recommended that those suffering from postpartum depression speak with family and friends, join a support group if available in their community, consult a medical or mental health professional, focus on their own well-being and that of their baby by eating healthy meals, maintaining a balanced diet, exercising, avoiding the use of alcohol, coffee, and cigarettes, and following the treatment recommended by their doctor and/or psychiatrist.

Postpartum Support International.

Phone: 800-944-4PPD (800-944-4773)

Website: http://www.postpartum.net

For information about treatment, support groups, and resources in the United States and 25 other countries.

Postpartum Education for Parents.

Phone: 805-967-7636 / Website: http://www.sbpep.org

A 24-hour support line is available for personal support, from basic infant care to baby blues and other perinatal topics. (This can be called long distance.)

1-800-311-BABY (1-800-311-2229)

En español: 800-504-7081 Para información sobre servicios prenatales en tu comunidad.

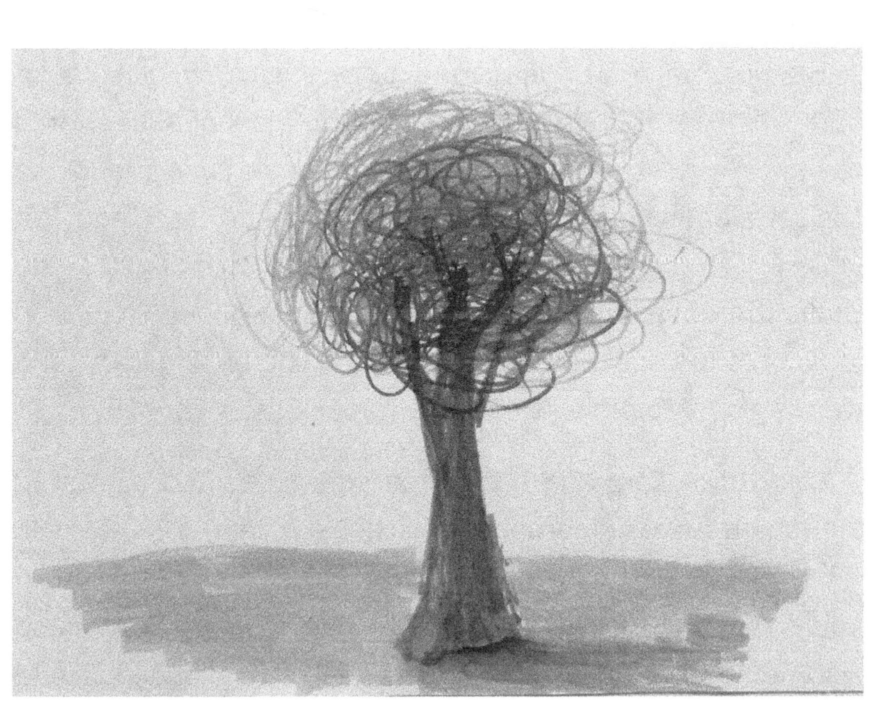

DR. MIGUEL HERNÁNDEZ

Alcohol-induced Depression

Sorrow Intoxicated by Fictitious Joy

Readers may wonder if the use of alcohol can cause depression, or if depression can lead to alcohol abuse. Both cases are true. However, in many scenarios, we face the clinical dilemma of what came first: the chicken or the egg. We believe it's crucial to educate the Hispanic community in the United States about this issue. The number of people turning to alcohol to cope with their sadness is increasing daily, and we want to help prevent this fake happiness.

Mood disorders and substance addiction often coexist in the United States (Journal of Clinical Psychiatry, 2006). While moderate alcohol consumption may not be harmful for most adults, about 18 million American adults have an alcohol use disorder that causes distress and harm (National Institute on Alcohol Abuse and Alcoholism). Annually, 88,000 people (62,000 men and 26,000 women) die from alcohol-related causes, making alcohol use the fourth leading preventable cause of death in the country. Additionally, in 2014, 31% of traffic fatalities in the United States were alcohol-related (National Center for Statistics and Analysis, 2015). Alcoholics are more likely to present with depressive symptoms and have a 9 to 22 times higher likelihood of suicide than non-alcoholics.

They are also more violent and more likely to attempt suicide in shorter periods of time (National Institute on Alcohol Abuse and Alcoholism).

According to the Dietary Guidelines for Americans, moderate alcohol consumption —defined as one drink per day for women and up to two drinks per day for men— has been promoted as beneficial for reducing the risk of mortality from heart problems, ischemic strokes, and diabetes. However, it's important to note that alcohol use, even in moderation, may not be safe for everyone. Individuals with a genetic predisposition to alcoholism, certain medical conditions, or those taking medications for medical or psychiatric issues may be at increased risk of harm. While the benefits of moderate alcohol consumption may be valid for some, it's essential to educate the population about its potential risks.

Adolescents with alcohol use disorder are at high risk for major depression, especially at a younger age. Studies suggest that the relationship between alcohol use and depression is bidirectional, with each problem contributing to the other (Addiction, 2016; Curr Addict Rep, 2016). In the DSM-IV statistical and diagnostic manual, alcohol-induced psychiatric disorders are classified into several categories, including delirium, dementia, amnestic disorder, psychotic disorder, mood disorder, anxiety disorder, sexual disorder, and sleep disorder. Alcohol-induced depression falls into the group of mood disorders induced by alcohol.

Alcohol-induced depression can cause a combination of classic symptoms from both disorders, as well as a history of alcohol abuse or dependence. However, it's essential to distinguish between major depression that leads to alcohol abuse and dependence, and alcohol-induced depression, which may disappear once the person stops drinking or receives successful treatment. The most frequent symptoms include a depressed mood, decreased interest in activities, sleep and psychomotor disturbances, fatigue, feelings of worthlessness, difficulty concentrating, and self-destructive or suicidal thoughts.

Alcohol acts as a depressant by reducing anxiety, inhibitions, and tension. This may make individuals feel relaxed and happy for a short period, leading them to believe that alcohol is good for their mental health. However, many people who drink alcohol as a refuge to hide their depression may develop an addiction that is difficult to control without professional help.

The treatment for alcohol-induced depression typically includes individual and group psychotherapies, such as Alcoholics Anonymous. However, in cases where the patient's life or the lives of others are at risk due to alcohol intoxication and dependence accompanied by depression, hospitalization with acute intervention may be necessary. Medications such as anxiolytics and antipsychotics can be used to help manage complications related to alcohol withdrawal syndrome.

At the outpatient and inpatient levels, various medications such as antidepressants, disulfiram, naltrexone, and benzodiazepines can be used to treat alcohol-induced depression. The goal of treatment is to achieve remission of the alcohol use disorder and, consequently, the disappearance of depression if it is exclusively induced by alcohol use. In alcoholics, depression has a better prognosis for improvement and can resolve more quickly with abstinence.

In conclusion, we recommend seeking help from a primary care physician, social worker, mental health counselor, psychologist, or psychiatrist if you experience the following situations:

- You feel sad and cannot stop drinking alcohol, or are drinking more than planned.

- You have symptoms of alcohol withdrawal, such as sweating, tremors, headache, or irritability when not drinking, or you need a drink in the mornings to avoid these symptoms.

- Your daily responsibilities are affected by alcohol use.

- You feel guilty about actions taken or not taken due to alcohol use.

- You have experienced loss of impulse control while under the influence of alcohol, have legal, marital, work, academic, or medical problems associated with alcohol use, or have suicidal thoughts or attempts.

Remember that alcohol is not a solution for difficult moments, feelings of anguish, or depression. In fact, it often adds to the problem and can lead down a path of destruction.

For information on alcohol, depression, and other mental illnesses:

1-866-615-NIMH (6464) (the call is free for those who live in the United States)

E-mail: nimhinfo@nih.gov

Website: http://www.nimh.nih.gov

(Drawing made by hand "The badly hurt and the sensitive")

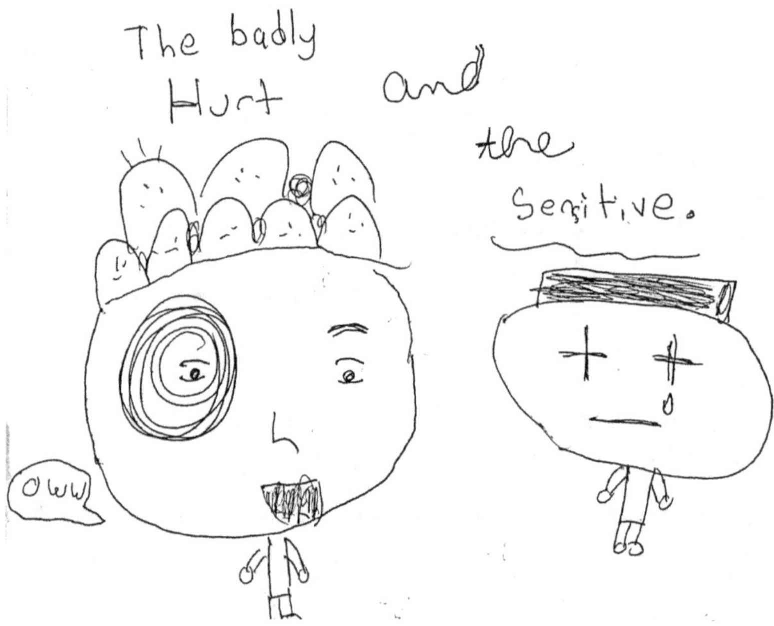

Bipolar Disorder

The Expected Experience of Extreme Highs and Lows

Bipolar disorder, also known as bipolar affective disorder, is a serious illness that has a significant impact on society. The consequences of this disorder can be dire, including suicide and economic losses due to prolonged absences from work, which can be longer than those associated with major depression. These findings were revealed in a study conducted by the National Institute of Mental Health of the United States (NIHM).

Unfortunately, many people are not aware of the disorder's etiology, symptomatology, risks, and treatment. It's common to hear someone say, "you're so bipolar" to describe a person who changes moods rapidly. People may also use the term "mania" to describe someone who engages in a particular behavior repeatedly, such as "that boy has a mania for touching that" or "I have a mania for touching my hair when I talk". However, it's important to note that the use of the words bipolar and mania in these contexts is incorrect, as bipolar refers to a psychiatric disorder and mania to a phase of bipolar illness. Therefore, it's essential to have a thorough understanding of the realities of this disorder.

When it comes to the causes of bipolar disorder, we now understand that there is a genetic predisposition to the disease. For instance, if you have a close relative with the condition, your likelihood of developing the disorder is at least 25 times higher than that of someone without affected family members.

According to the DSM-IV, the manual used by psychiatrists to diagnose mental disorders, there are two types of bipolar disorder: bipolar disorder type I and bipolar disorder type II. The main difference between the two types is primarily in the combination of episodes that each present. Bipolar disorder type I is characterized by at least one episode of mania, with or without an episode of major depression, or with the presence of both. In contrast, bipolar disorder type II is characterized by episodes of depression alternating with episodes of hypomania. Now that we have an idea of the classification of bipolar disorders, it is important to understand what we mean when we talk about episodes of mania or hypomania.

A manic episode, or mania, is typically characterized by a period of at least one week of irritability or elevated mood that significantly impairs social and occupational functioning. During this period, at least three of the following symptoms must also be present: grandiosity, decreased need for sleep, rapid speech, easy distractibility, increased psychomotor activity or engaging in many activities at once, and excessive involvement in pleasurable activities. These episodes cannot be caused by a physical condition or be induced by substance use. Similarly, a hypomanic episode has the same symptoms as a manic episode, but with a few differences: its duration is four days instead of one week, and the decrease in social and occupational functioning is not as pronounced. Therefore, many people with type II are not diagnosed in time, as they can function relatively well in society without needing to be hospitalized.

When it comes to treatment, the good news is that despite being a chronic condition with fluctuations and relapses, there are appropriate treatments for both acute and non-acute stages. During the acute stages, especially in type I bipolar disorder, hospitalization and the use of antipsychotic drugs and benzodiazepines are almost always necessary. For maintenance treatment and relapse prevention, lithium salts and anticonvulsant agents such as valproic acid, carbamazepine, gabapentin, and lamotrigine are used. In recent years, atypical antipsychotic drugs have also been approved for this stage of treatment. Additionally, it's important to note that psychotherapy is one of the most important tools in almost all phases of therapeutic intervention for bipolar disorder.

Lastly, to prevent relapse episodes, it's important for patients to commit to taking their medication as prescribed, attending regular medical visits, and participating in educational psychotherapy. Family involvement and support throughout the disease process, as well as participation in community prevention programs, can also improve the chances of success.

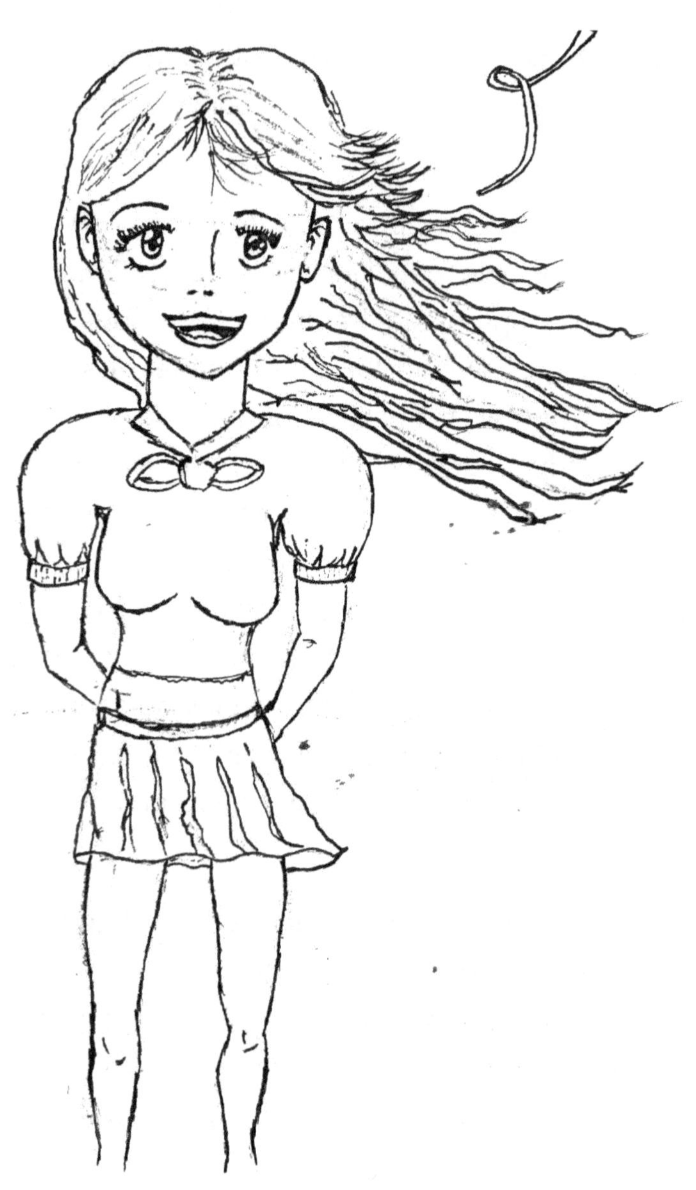

Schizophrenia

The Improbable Sanity of a Fractured Reality

One percent of the population is affected by schizophrenia at some point in their lives. Schizophrenic patients occupy more hospital beds than any other patient with a mental illness (Psychiatry, Janis L. Cutler, 2010). Despite being one of the most well-studied and described mental disorders, schizophrenia still has a devastating social and economic impact. The social stigma of mental disorders, often negatively fueled by the press, radio, and television, continues to influence the deterioration and undesirable progression of the disease. Therefore, we believe it is important to share information about an illness characterized by complex rifts in reality and embedded in a world fragmented by an unrealistic sanity.

The term schizophrenia was coined by the psychiatrist Eugen Bleuer in 1911, but as early as 1856, the German psychiatrist Emil Kraepelin referred to the condition using the term "Dementia Praecoux" or "domentia praecox," to describe a deteriorating illness affecting the young population. The word schizophrenia is derived from the Greek "skhizen", meaning "to separate," and "phren," meaning "mind," reflecting the concept that in schizophrenia, there is a separation of the mind from reality.

Schizophrenia affects both males and females equally, with onset occurring earlier in males than in females. Interestingly, statistical research has shown that individuals who develop schizophrenia are more likely to have been born in the winter or early spring months. In the United States, those born between the months of January and April have a higher risk of developing the disease (Kaplan and Sadock's Synopsis of Psychiatry by Benjamin J. Sadock, 11th edition, 2014).

Schizophrenia is characterized by changes in thinking, perception, and behavior. According to the DSM-IV (Diagnostic and Statistical Manual of Mental Disorders), it is a disorder where there are two or more of the following symptoms for at least one month: hallucinations or delusions (perceptions not based on reality), delusions (of persecution or grandeur), disorganized behavior or speech, apathetic expression or altered emotional expression, lack of motivation or loss of verbal expression. All of these symptoms must cause significant impairment in occupational and social functioning for at least six months, and cannot be caused by the use of alcohol, illicit substances, or medical illness. If the impairment is present for less than six months, it is referred to as schizophreniform disorder.

We should understand that not all psychotic disorders are schizophrenia, as there are other disorders with very similar presentations that could be confused with schizophrenia, such as schizoaffective disorder, drug-induced psychotic disorder, bipolar disorder with psychosis, and any type of delirium.

There are several types of schizophrenia. For example, the paranoid type is characterized by thoughts of persecution, suspicion, and distrust. The patient may believe that aliens are planning to poison them or that the government is controlling them remotely by satellite. The disorganized type may present with disorganized behavior and speech and with neglect of personal hygiene, and it is common among many of the homeless individuals we see on the streets who are abandoned, without shelter, and unkempt. The catatonic type may present with rigidity, negativism, and the affected person may adopt the same body posture for a long time. Other types include residual or undifferentiated types.

Although the cause of schizophrenia is still unknown, It is believed to be the result of a combination of genetic and environmental factors. Studies of twins and families of patients have shown that there is a high genetic contribution to the development of the disease. Additionally, environmental factors such as stressful life situations, low socioeconomic status, and viral infections during pregnancy have been associated with the onset of this mental disorder.

Another important factor is that individuals with schizophrenia tend to smoke more cigarettes, drink more alcohol, and use more illicit drugs than the general population. This behavior is due to their impaired decision-making ability and to alleviate the uncomfortable and bothersome symptoms of the disease.

Despite the unknown cause, the good news is that there is treatment available for this disease. Antipsychotic agents such as haloperidol, olanzapine, risperidone, and clozapine, to name a few, in conjunction with psychotherapy, can control the disease and may decrease relapses, which are common in schizophrenia. Patients must remain compliant with their treatment and attend regular medical appointments to ensure, albeit often slowly, their reintegration and optimal functioning in society.

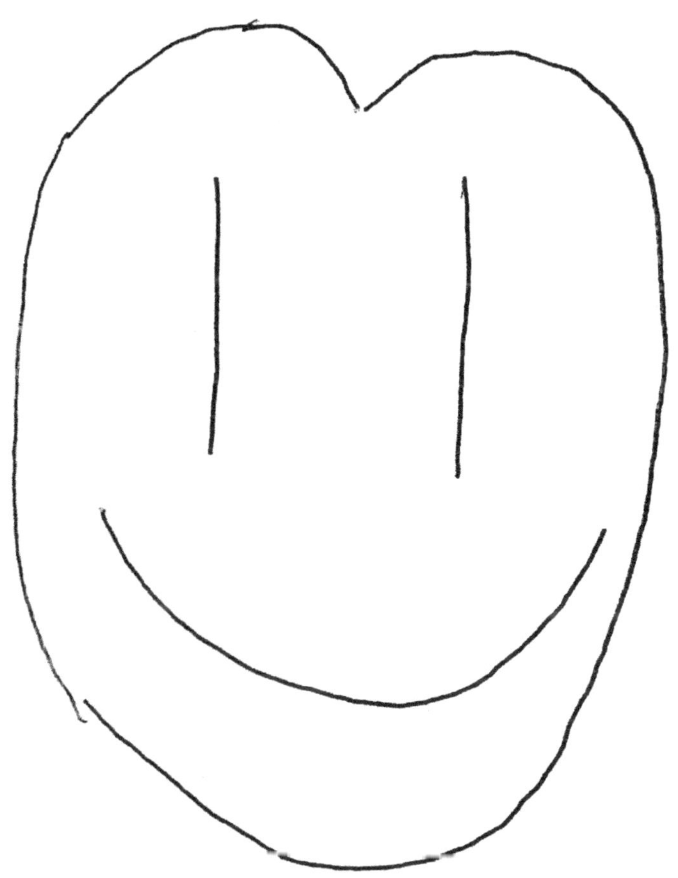

Post-Traumatic Stress Disorder

A Loyal Testimony of Survival

According to the National Institute of Mental Health (NIMH), approximately 7.7 million individuals aged 18 and older experience post-traumatic stress disorder (PTSD) in a given year, as referenced in an article published in the Archives of General Psychiatry in June 2005. In our lives, we all face the risk of exposure to catastrophic events that could result in becoming victims or witnesses of highly dangerous situations. The increase of global wars, terrorist attacks, and natural disasters not only increases the real possibility of such events but also the perception of vulnerability to them. It's essential to understand the causes, symptoms, and treatment of PTSD, which for those who suffer from it, goes beyond just a faithful testimony of survival.

Post-traumatic stress disorder is a set of symptoms that can occur as an immediate or delayed response to a catastrophic life event. Some of the most common events that can trigger this disorder include war experiences, terrorist attacks, traffic accidents, natural disasters, sexual assault, physical or sexual abuse, or any situation in which one's life was in danger, or where one witnessed others' lives being endangered, or significant injury or death occurring.

Interestingly, not everyone reacts in the same way or develops typical symptoms of PTSD after exposure to catastrophic or dangerous situations. Certain individuals have risk factors that increase the likelihood of developing this condition when exposed to or having experienced traumatic or undesirable events. These risk factors include being female, having a history of depression or anxiety, experiencing separation from parents during childhood, and having a history of antisocial behavior

According to the Diagnostic and Statistical Manual of Psychiatry, Fourth Edition (DSM-IV), there are approximately five main manifestations that characterize this disorder. Firstly, it is necessary to have been exposed to a traumatic event and to have responded to that event with intense feelings of fear, hopelessness, and horror. Secondly, the event is persistently re-experienced in different ways, such as through dreams, intrusive thoughts, images, or any internal or external stimuli that symbolize the traumatic experience, among others. In the same order, there is a behavior of rejection or avoidance of everything related to the place or things associated with the event. For example, people may avoid traveling by car if they had a traffic accident, or they may not go out in the street if they were victims of a mugging or rape. Many times, people do not remember important parts of the event. Additionally, people may persistently suffer from symptoms not present before the incident, such as difficulty sleeping and concentrating, hypervigilance, irritability, and exaggerated response to situations of less danger but similar to the traumatic event. Finally, the duration of symptoms should be at least one month and should cause significant distress socially, at work, or in other important areas of the individual.

There are various forms of treatment available for post-traumatic stress disorder, including both pharmacological and non-pharmacological approaches. Pharmacological treatments involve medication such as antidepressants, anxiolytics, beta-blockers, and mood stabilizers. Non-pharmacological treatments include cognitive, behavioral, psychodynamic, and hypnotherapeutic psychotherapy.

It is important to note that post-traumatic stress disorder can affect anyone in the population, not just war veterans. Many Hispanic people may be suffering from this disorder, but may feel embarrassed or lack knowledge about it. We encourage them to talk to their primary care physician, psychologists, social workers, psychiatrists, or anyone in the mental health sector about their traumatic experiences and their symptoms, as seeking help can make a significant difference in their lives.

Mental Health and Physical Activity

Allies for Your Well-Being

It's common for patients to wonder why they're advised to exercise regularly, particularly aerobic exercise, in addition to eating healthily during psychiatric consultations. Concerns about limited time, low income to pay for a gym, chronic pain, or medical conditions can add to the challenges. Individuals with serious mental health conditions are at a higher risk for physical illnesses, metabolic syndrome, diabetes, and cardiovascular conditions. Although genetic factors play a role in these disorders, lifestyle, and environmental factors, such as smoking, obesity, inappropriate diet, and low physical activity, also have a significant impact (BMC Psychiatry. 2014).

Therefore, we want to emphasize the importance of physical activity and mental health, which are interconnected for overall well-being. We hope this information will be helpful for our readers.

Improving one's overall health condition can lower the risk of developing mental illness. Aerobic exercise has been shown to reduce symptoms of depression and anxiety. Exercise is beneficial for these illnesses because it improves energy levels, concentration, and sleep, which are crucial factors for mental well-being (NAMI.org). Additionally, there is evidence to suggest that exercise can prevent the development of depression.

You may be wondering how exercise can help with mental illness. According to the American Psychological Association, studies on animals since 1980 have shown that exercise increases the concentration of norepinephrine in brain regions related to stress response, beyond the monoaminergic theory. For many experts, it's not just about increasing levels of norepinephrine, which is largely produced in an area of the brain called the locus coeruleus. It's a complex biological mechanism in which exercise gives the body the opportunity to cope with stress by inducing physiological stress response systems to communicate with each other. This includes a more harmonious communication between the cardiovascular, muscular, renal, and immune systems, with two protagonists: the central nervous system and the sympathetic nervous system. They refine their physiological language to improve future responses to stress.

The U.S. Department of Health and Human Services recommends that children between the ages of 6 and 17 engage in at least 60 minutes of physical activity per day, consisting of moderate or vigorous aerobic exercise, along with bone and muscle strengthening activities at least twice a week. For adults, the guidelines suggest engaging in at least 150 minutes (2.5 hours) of moderate-intensity aerobic exercise per week, in addition to performing stretching exercises twice a week such as push-ups, weightlifting, and more.

Many people find gym memberships too expensive, but you don't need a gym to get active. Taking a walk, run, or bike ride are all great options. And don't forget simple steps like taking the stairs instead of the elevator or parking farther away to walk to your destination, which can boost your physical activity in a beneficial way.

Patients with psychiatric illnesses, such as schizophrenia and bipolar disorder, who are typically treated with antipsychotics or mood stabilizers, have a higher risk of developing obesity and metabolic syndrome.

It may be helpful for psychiatric units to incorporate vigorous aerobic and stretching exercises into their therapeutic routines for patients without contraindications. However, there may be legal and medical-psychiatric risks that limit the use of this approach during hospitalization.

As more studies are conducted, it is increasingly believed that exercise can be just as beneficial as antidepressants in certain cases. However, it's important to view exercise as a preventive and supportive tool for maintaining good mental health and improving pre-existing mental conditions. While exercise can be a helpful addition to traditional psychiatric treatments, it should not be seen as a replacement without proper medical supervision. In fact, substituting exercise for psychiatric treatment without proper supervision can often result in a decline in mental health, prolonging the suffering of those affected and significantly increasing the risk of psychiatric complications.

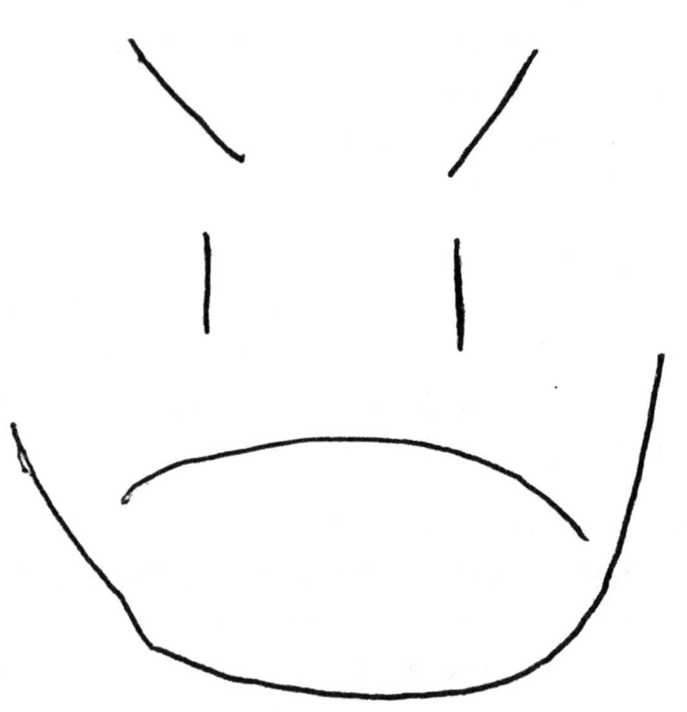

Psychotherapy in Psychiatric Treatment
The Art of Healing Communication

Special thanks to Dr. Kelania Jiménez MA, MHC for her contributions.

As we all know, psychiatry is a highly specialized field that provides extensive knowledge about human behavior. One of its primary goals is to evaluate, diagnose, and treat individuals in order to help them recover. In psychiatric treatment, there are two fundamental modalities that continue to evolve: the biological modality and the psychotherapeutic modality. While both modalities are important, psychotherapy has become an increasingly valuable tool for addressing a wide range of mental health issues and promoting overall well-being.

Psychotherapy is a process of communication between a therapist and a patient aimed at improving the patient's quality of life through changes in behavior, attitude, affect, and thinking. By interacting with the therapist, the patient can express their ideas, emotions, and feelings. Meanwhile, the therapist evaluates the patient's needs and tries to effect change through the therapeutic process. During the initial session, the clinician and patient develop a relationship centered around building empathy and understanding the circumstances or reasons that led to the patient seeking help. Then, a thorough assessment is conducted, which involves gathering personal and biographical information to develop the patient's medical history. After this, the clinician and patient can discuss the demands and expectations of the therapy, including the conditions, responsibilities, approximate duration, and steps of the therapeutic approach.

While psychotherapy can be a powerful tool for addressing mental health issues, it's important to consider various patient variables that go beyond the clinical diagnosis. These may include personality traits, family dynamics, and environmental factors.

In most forms of psychotherapy, and particularly in psychoanalysis, memory work is essential. The goal is to recover and elaborate on memories by linking them with present-day experiences that can alter the way the memory is consolidated. Recollection and free association are fundamental components of any treatment, as they allow patients to explore their thoughts and express everything that comes to mind. The interpretation of these elements enables different emotional connections to be established. Confrontational comments are particularly important in building these connections.

Similarly, resistance, transference, and countertransference are all present in psychotherapy. Resistance refers to any attitude that opposes the therapeutic framework and hinders access to the contents of the patient's unconscious. This can include opposition to the therapist, which may have either positive or negative connotations. Transference is a psychoanalytic process or psychological mechanism through which a person unconsciously transfers and reactivates old, repressed emotions, expectations, or subtle desires in their new social relationships. Countertransference, on the other hand, refers to the repressed feelings of the psychotherapist related to their past experiences, which are often manifested to the patient unconsciously and may result in prejudices or inappropriate predispositions that could lead to therapeutic failure

Increasing the patient's awareness of their illness is a fundamental principle of psychotherapy, as it enables the patient to become conscious of what is not easily visible, since it is retained in their unconscious. In this sense, the therapist's main objective is to help the patient recognize their problems and thus begin a journey towards emotional well-being.

There is scientific evidence that supports the effectiveness of psychotherapy. A study conducted by George Y. Ankuta and Norman Abeles on patients at the Michigan State University Psychology Clinic, titled "Client Satisfaction, Clinical Significance, and Meaningful Change in Psychotherapy," demonstrated that patients who participated in psychotherapy reported higher levels of satisfaction and improvement compared to a control group. Similarly, a study conducted in Scotland called "The Effectiveness of Counseling" showed that counseling or psychotherapy is a clinically effective intervention, as it reduces psychiatric hospitalizations by helping individuals achieve better mental health.

Psychotherapy plays a critical and indispensable role in the treatment of psychiatric disorders. Numerous studies have shown that psychotherapy is more effective than certain types of interventions and can significantly reduce symptoms of mental disorders such as major depression and anxiety disorders.

The need to connect with others is essential to human existence. In psychotherapy, effective communication is key to building a strong relationship between the therapist and patient. Empathy, acceptance, and clear communication are fundamental aspects of this relationship. The therapist plays an important role as a mediator and collaborator, working with the patient to promote emotional and mental well-being. Seeing positive changes in patients is incredibly rewarding for therapists, and it's why we do what we do. Every therapist has their own style and approach, but our goal is always the same: to help our patients achieve their optimal level of functioning and well-being.

CHAPTER III:

Other Psychiatric Disorders and Topics of Interest

Dementia

Agony of Memories in the Sad Twilight of Forgetfulness

Dementia is derived from the Latin word meaning "far from the mind". It is not a disease itself but rather a syndrome that can have various origins. Although Alzheimer's disease is the most common cause of dementia, accounting for more than half of all cases, it is not the only cause. There is a general misconception, especially in Hispanic culture, that aging is synonymous with dementia, but this is not true. According to information presented at the International Conference on Alzheimer's Disease (ICAD), Hispanics with Alzheimer's disease tend to consult physicians later, even though they experience symptoms of dementia seven years earlier than non-Hispanics. More concerning is that 40% of Hispanics in the United States with dementia are undiagnosed and untreated. The annual cost of dementia in the United States is approximately $150 billion. Therefore, it is vital to share information about this condition, which shrouds the memories of those who suffer from it in shadows of agony, and leads them, in living bodies without memory, into the sad penumbra of oblivion.

Aloysius "Alois" Alzheimer, a psychiatrist and neuropathologist, was the first to publish a case of dementia in 1906. He defined it as a progressive and fatal cognitive disorder that impairs neurons, causing difficulties with memory, language, thinking, and behavior. It's important to note that dementia involves neuronal damage, which results in behavioral changes beyond those attributable to normal aging, and is not limited to memory loss alone.

The exact cause or etiology of Alzheimer's disease is still not fully understood, but it is believed to be multifactorial, and still under investigation and debate. Factors such as age, diet, environment, and genetics are thought to play a role. Specifically, the accumulation of senile plaques and neurofibrillary tangles in neurons, associated with mutations of multiple genes, have been linked to the origin and development of Alzheimer's disease. Some of the genes believed to be involved in this process include the amyloid precursor protein, located on the long arm of chromosome 21, presenilin 1 and 2, apolipoprotein E, among others. Hispanics have also shown a modest relationship with mutations in chromosomes 10q/12p, and a strong relationship in chromosome 18q (Lee and Mayeux, 2006) (8).

Likewise, there are risk factors associated with Alzheimer's disease, including being female, Hispanic (seven times more likely), a history of head trauma (three to four times more likely), low education, Down syndrome, having relatives affected by Alzheimer's, and metabolic syndrome (high blood pressure, abdominal obesity, high glucose, and abnormal blood lipid levels).

The disease is diagnosed clinically based on the patient's history, taken from both the patient and their relatives, and on the patient's behavior. Blood tests and imaging studies can be used to exclude other diseases with similar manifestations and symptoms. The definitive diagnosis is made by identifying typical lesions or markers of the disease through histopathological studies after the affected person's death.

Alzheimer's disease affects the most important areas of cognitive function, such as memory, language, attention, orientation, and problem-solving skills. It starts with forgetting the names of friends, family members, and the location of personal items such as keys. As the disease progresses, patients may forget significant parts of their personal history, even getting lost in their own neighborhood or home. Alzheimer's dementia is progressive and has different stages, ranging from very mild dysfunction (stages one and two) that may go unnoticed by the patient and others, to severe difficulties (stages six and seven) where the patient loses language and only remembers their name. In advanced stages, they lose the ability to perform basic activities of daily living such as eating, bathing, and laughing, and eventually lose contact with reality.

Unfortunately, there is still no cure for the disease. However, there are relief management options for patients and their families, ranging from the use of medications such as donepezil, galantamine, memantine, rivastigmine, tacrine, etc., to psychotherapies and special care for the patient. Although there is no definitive evidence to support a specific diet or preventive measure for the disease, it is recommended to reduce modifiable risk factors mentioned earlier such as high blood pressure, high blood glucose (sugar), and high cholesterol. It's worth noting that these factors can be favorably modified by lifestyle changes and following a healthy diet.

Finally, we will share some recommendations for family members, friends, or caregivers of patients with Alzheimer's disease, extracted from the website of the Alzheimer's Association:

- Monitor any discomfort (pain, hunger, sleep, infection, fatigue, full bladder, room temperature).

- Ensure good sleep habits (early exposure to light, daily exercise, avoid medication before bed, fixed meal times).

- Avoid confronting or arguing with them about the truth.

- Redirect them by being flexible and patient.

- Create a calm and simple environment.

- Allow them to have good rest.

- Provide safe objects and respect their modesty.

- Secure the doors with locks and remove weapons from their reach.

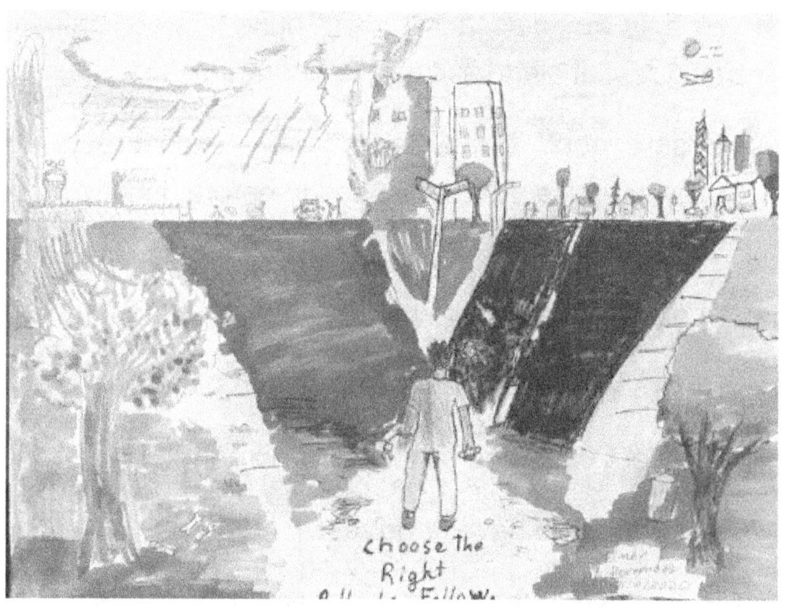

Choose the
Right
Follow.

Domestic Violence

The Ignored Warning of a Tragedy

Domestic violence is the most common cause of nonfatal injury to women in the United States, affecting women of all races, religions, and social strata (NEJM, 1999; Kaplan and Sadock's Synopsis of Psychiatry by Benjamin J Sadock 11th, 2014). It is estimated that 2 to 4 million women are abused by their intimate partners each year (JAMA, 1992). In the Hispanic media in the USA, reports of domestic violence cases are increasingly frequent, often leading to tragic outcomes. It is important to raise awareness about domestic violence, which can be an insidious and underestimated sign of misfortune.

Domestic violence is not limited to men abusing women; it also occurs, albeit less frequently, in cases where women abuse men. It affects same-sex relationships as well.

omen who are at an increased risk of injury due to domestic violence include those whose partners abuse alcohol or use drugs, are unemployed, have less than a high school education, or are ex-husbands or ex-boyfriends (NEJM, 1999).

It's important for women to be aware that abusive men

often come from families where they were abused as children or witnessed parental abuse. These partners are usually immature, dependent, and suffer from strong feelings of inadequacy. Additionally, 50% of battered women grew up in violent homes and have dependent-type personality characteristics (Kaplan and Sadock's Synopsis of Psychiatry by Benjamin J Sadock, 11th edition, 2014).

It is alarming that domestic violence can become a cycle where the act itself becomes a stimulant and the abuser is much more likely to repeat the abuse again. But the question is: why do so many people commit acts of domestic violence against their partners, whom they should love and protect? The dynamics behind it can be diverse, but they may include identification with the aggressor, whether it's the abusive parent or boss, the need to test the partner's limits to prove love, or distorted desires to express masculinity. At times, the abuse can be a displacement of the aggression that others have inflicted on their lives.

Victims of abuse may experience a range of behaviors from their abusers, including control of finances, emotional manipulation, intimidation, isolation from family and friends, abandonment, rape, forced sexual contact, sexist comments, harassment, neglect, jealousy, possessive acts, deprivation of physical and economic resources, and restriction of medical and dental care sought, as well as threats to harm family and/ or friends, take away children, harm animals, use weapons, or commit murder. All of these behaviors can lead to a loss of self-esteem, depression, insomnia, anxiety, feelings of hopelessness, emotional numbness, and other mental health disorders.

Family therapy, in combination with support from social and legal agencies, may help the abuser control their violent impulses. However, it is also important to always have a safety plan when in a domestic violence situation.

- The safety plan should include:

- Identifying a safe place to go.

- Avoiding rooms without exits or with weapons, such as bathrooms and kitchens.

- Memorizing important phone numbers.

- Establishing signs and codes with family and friends to signal for help.

- Knowing what to say or do if the abuser becomes violent.

Finally, I want to emphasize that if you are a victim or have been a victim of domestic violence, it is crucial to act quickly and intelligently to protect your life, as well as the lives of your children and family members. We must also remember that no relationship should ever take priority over individual integrity and freedom.

For more information about domestic violence, please visit http://www.ncadv.org

If you need immediate help, please call 911 or The National Domestic Violence Hotline at 1-800-799-SAFE (7233).

Fibromyalgia

Chronic Waves of Pain in a Psychoneurobiological Ocean

One might ask why a psychiatrist is discussing fibromyalgia. The controversy surrounding the cause, symptoms, and treatment of fibromyalgia is not limited to patients who are often overwhelmed by tides of chronic and insidious pain, but also continues to cause debates among rheumatologists, neurologists, pain specialists, and psychiatrists. Fibromyalgia is described as a disorder of the central nervous system caused by neurobiological abnormalities that result in physiological and emotional pain, cognitive failure, and physical and neuropsychological symptoms (Galvez-Sanchez, C. M., Duschek, S., & Reyes Del Paso, G. A. 2019). The approach to therapy and the ultimate truth of the etiology of the disease seem to depend on the specialist's perspective. The psychosocial repercussions of this disease and its comorbidities are devastating for individuals who suffer from it. Therefore, it is crucial to delve into the subject of fibromyalgia, an ocean of deep and rough waters with psychosomatic swells.

According to the American Pain Society (APS), fibromyalgia affects more than five million people in the United States, making it one of the most common chronic pain conditions. Although fibromyalgia was first described in the 1800s, it was not until 1976 that it became known as fibromyalgia, replacing the earlier term "fibrositis" (Inanici F, Yunus MB, 2004). The name derives from the Latin "fibro," referring to fibrous tissue, ligaments, and tendons, and the Greek "myo" and "algos," which mean muscle and pain, respectively.

Fibromyalgia occurs in 2% of the population, across all ethnic groups and cultures, and affects women more than men, with a ratio of 8:1 (Levenson, psychosomatic medicine, 2007) (13). The most common age of onset is between 30 and 50 years old, although it can affect children and the elderly. Fibromyalgia is more prevalent in people with low socioeconomic and educational levels, and it is 50% more common in semi-skilled or unskilled workers than in professionals (White et al., 1999).

The precise cause of fibromyalgia has not been established, but current medical evidence suggests that a combination of environmental factors and individual vulnerability can initiate a biopsychosocial process that leads to the development of the disease. Genetic risk factors, psychological risk factors such as abuse and maltreatment in childhood or adulthood, and social risk factors such as low social and educational levels have been associated with fibromyalgia. Biological precipitating factors such as infections, including those caused by Epstein Barr virus, Q fever, viral meningitis, and hepatitis, as well as neck trauma, have also been described. Psychosocial precipitants such as periods of significant stress, perpetuating factors such as chronic infections, sleep disorders, autoimmune diseases, neuroendocrine changes such as increased substance P in the cerebrospinal fluid (Rusell et al., 1994), and psychological perpetuating factors, including depression and perception or belief of illness, can all contribute to the development and maintenance of fibromyalgia.

It is believed that fibromyalgia patients experience central sensitization due to nerve stimulation, which causes abnormality in brain neurotransmitters, leading to a lowered pain threshold. Pain receptors develop a memory to pain, making them more sensitive to it (Mayo Clinic, 2020).

Fibromyalgia cannot be diagnosed through blood, urine, or imaging tests. The American College of Rheumatology (ACR) established diagnostic criteria in 1990 which includes widespread pain lasting for at least 3 months and pain in 11 of 18 specific body sites. The pain should occur above and below the waist and on both sides of the body. Common points of pain are the neck, middle and upper back, shoulders, upper chest, hips, and knees. Individuals with fibromyalgia experience an increased sensitivity to painful stimuli known as hyperalgesia and pain in response to non-painful stimuli known as allodynia. As a result, many individuals with fibromyalgia feel pain even with a hug or holding hands with someone. In addition, fibromyalgia causes problems with thinking and memory, commonly referred to as Fibro Fog, as well as menstrual cramps and morning stiffness.

People with fibromyalgia may also have coexisting conditions such as chronic fatigue syndrome, depression, anxiety, endometriosis, panic and post-traumatic stress disorder, headaches, and irritable bowel syndrome.

When it comes to managing and treating fibromyalgia, it's important for patients to understand the need for a multidisciplinary therapeutic approach that includes psychiatric follow-up without stigmatizing mental health. It is recommended that a team consisting of a primary care physician, rheumatologist, pain specialist, neurologist, and psychiatrist work together to treat the condition. Patients should be educated about the risks of self-medication, particularly with analgesics and narcotics, and the importance of seeking out both conventional and alternative therapies.

Psychotherapies, such as cognitive and behavioral therapy combined with exercise, have been shown to be the most beneficial. Support groups and ongoing counseling through educational resources are also crucial. Practices like meditation, relaxation, yoga, Qi Gong, lymphatic drainage therapy, balneotherapy, deep breathing, tai chi, visualization exercises, healthy diet, optimal sleep, and aerobic exercise should be part of multidisciplinary management.

Serotonin reuptake inhibitors and tricyclic antidepressant medications have been found to be helpful, as many patients also experience depression and anxiety. Antidepressants improve the pain threshold. The US Food and Drug Administration has approved pregabalin (Lyrica), duloxetine (Cymbalta), and milnacipran (Savella) for the treatment of fibromyalgia. There is no evidence of benefit in using non-steroidal anti-inflammatory drugs (e.g., naproxen, ibuprofen, aspirin) when used alone. The use of narcotic opioids (codeine, oxycodone, hydromorphone) and benzodiazepines, such as alprazolam, clonazepam, and diazepam, has a risk of addiction. Tramadol, acetaminophen, gabapentin, and muscle relaxants have been effective in pain management.

If you want more information on fibromyalgia and other mental illnesses, you can contact the National Institute of Mental Health (NIMH) by calling 1-866-615-NIMH (6464) toll-free within the United States, emailing nimhinfo@nih.gov, or visiting their website at http://www.nimh.nih.gov

Special thanks to Dr. Casilda Balmaceda, board-certified neurologist, for providing material on this topic.

Internet Addiction

Trapped in the Web

The internet is a valuable tool for work, education, information, entertainment, and leisure, and has become almost indispensable for most people worldwide. As psychiatrists, we never imagined during our medical training that technological advancements in communication and digital entertainment, including the significant use of cell phones, iPads, tablets, emails, video games, chat rooms, interactive instant messaging apps, and social networks such as Facebook, Twitter, Instagram, Facetime, Tango, and WhatsApp, could have addictive properties and the risk of abuse. Today, we consider internet addiction a mental disorder, comparable to abuse and dependence on licit and illicit substances such as alcohol, marijuana, and cocaine. It is crucial to provide guidance to the Hispanic community in the United States and around the world on this issue, as the number of individuals trapped by internet use is increasing, and many do not know how to break free or are not even aware that they are ensnared in the network.

The issue of internet addiction is relatively new. In 1996, Dr. Kimberly Young, an expert in internet addiction, first brought attention to the issue with a clinical report on a case of internet addiction. Since then, research on internet overuse and addiction has increased, including discussion of subtypes of internet-related problems such as online pornography, internet gambling, and video game addiction.

Although it is not included as a disorder in the DSM-V (Diagnostic and Statistical Manual of Mental Disorders, Fifth Edition), internet addiction has become a worldwide issue that can be defined as a non-chemical behavioral addiction involving machine-human interaction (Cerniglia L, Neuroscience and Biobehavioral Reviews, 2016).

The prevalence of internet addiction varies depending on culture and society, ranging from 6% to 15% of internet users, with rates increasing to 13% to 18.4% among college students (Young, Internet Addiction, 2011). This evidence supports the inclusion of internet addiction in the sixth edition of the DSM-VI (Indian J Public Health, 2015).

Certain factors may make individuals more vulnerable to addiction, such as low life satisfaction, a lack of strong social connections, low self-confidence, loss of hope, and dissatisfaction with important areas of their lives. While it has not been proven whether depression causes internet addiction or whether internet addiction causes depression, research has found a high correlation between the two syndromes (Peele, 1985; Young, 2011).

Low self-esteem and difficulties in family and school have been identified as factors associated with internet addiction

(Munno D, Psychiatry Res. 2016). Moreover, recent studies have found that being male, having attention deficit disorder, or experiencing deteriorating symptoms of other psychiatric disorders can also be risk factors for internet addiction (Psychiatry Clin Neurosci. 2016).

An interesting finding that demonstrates the negative impact of internet addiction is that adolescents with internet addiction have an increased risk of alcohol abuse and cigarette smoking (Lee BH Acta Paediatr. 2016).

Regarding neurobiological etiology, dopamine has been associated with internet addiction, specifically in the mesolimbic system, medial forebrain bundle (MFB), and endogenous opioid peptide system (ENK) (Di Chiara, 2000). Studies have found reduced white and gray matter in the orbitofrontal area of the cerebral cortex in individuals addicted to video games (Weng, Chuan-Bu 2013), as well as a smaller dorsolateral frontal cortex, rostral anterior cingulate cortex, and cerebellum (Yuan, K.; et al. (2011). Yang, Shaolin, ed.).

Dr. Young and Echeburua have identified warning signs that indicate dependence on information and communication technologies (ICT) or social networks, reflecting an Internet addiction. These signs are:

1. Sleep deprivation (<5 hours) due to excessive time spent connected to the network.

2. Neglecting important activities such as contact with family, social relationships, study, or health care.

3. Receiving complaints about network usage from someone close, such as parents or siblings.

4. Constantly thinking about the network, even when not connected, and feeling excessively irritated when the connection fails or is slow.

5. Failing to limit connection time and losing track of time.

6. Lying about actual time spent online or playing a video game.

7. Social isolation, irritability, and poor academic performance.

8. Feeling abnormal euphoria and activation when using the computer.

The Internet Addiction Diagnostic Questionnaire (IADQ) was the first diagnostic tool created in 1998, and the Internet Addiction Test (IAT) was the first validated instrument for assessing internet addiction (Widyanto, 2004; Young, 2011). Other useful instruments include the Internet Addiction Scale and the Internet Compulsive Use Risk Scale. The Brief Internet Game Screen (BIGS) Survey, which is available online at www.surveymonkey.com, is another instrument for screening internet game addiction.

According to CYAND (China Youth Association for Network Development) in its 2005 report, an individual should be classified as an Internet addict if they meet one of the following three conditions: feels that it is easier to achieve self-actualization online than in real life, feels dysphoria or depression every time the Internet does not work or its use stops, or tries to hide the actual time of use from family members or close people. A neuropsychological etiological model has been proposed, in which the main concept is that human beings have an instinct to seek pleasure and avoid pain. As a result, people continue to use the internet in order to achieve the same euphoric state, which gradually changes the euphoria into a habit with an episode of existential emptiness. Tolerance is produced, and more time is needed to reach the same level of pleasure. Shortly after, the physical and psychological syndrome of dependence appears. Once the use of the internet stops or decreases, the patient begins to feel lack of sleep, emotional instability, irritability, among other symptoms. At this stage, if the person is confronted, he/she shows frustration and begins to experience adverse effects around him/her, such as arguments, lying, fatigue, and social isolation.

To prevent Internet addiction, Ramón-Cortés (2010) suggests the following strategies:

- Limit device use and agree on computer hours.

- Foster relationships with other people.

- Encourage hobbies such as reading, watching movies, and participating in cultural activities.

- Promote sports and team activities.

- Develop group activities, such as volunteering, to stimulate communication and dialogue within the family.

Limiting the time spent online during childhood and adolescence (no more than 1.5-2 hours per day, except for weekends), locating computers in common areas such as the living room, and controlling content are important strategies to prevent internet addiction (Mayorgas, 2009; Enrique Echeburúa, 2010).

Some authors do not consider internet addiction as a disorder, but rather suggest that it is related to specific online content such as sex, gambling, or betting. They argue that the internet is used as a psycho-technological crutch that offers a more comfortable, less shameful, and less risky alternative to the behavior involved in satisfying specific real-life addictions, such as seeking prostitutes or gambling at a casino (Orzack & Orzack, 1999; Davis, 2001).

When it comes to treating internet addiction, there is little information available on psychotherapeutic approaches. One of the most commonly used treatments has been cognitive behavioral psychotherapy (CBT) in 12 sessions, which has yielded good results. It has also been combined with electroacupuncture. Other psychotherapy options include interpersonal therapy, structured cognitive therapy, and family therapy.

In terms of medication, bupropion (Wellbutrin) and escitalopram (Lexapro) have been effective in treating and managing internet game addiction, with bupropion being slightly more effective (Song J Psychiatry Clin Neurosci. 2016).

In conclusion, treating Internet addiction is a difficult and challenging task because many individuals refuse to acknowledge that they have an addiction problem. They justify their excessive or pathological use of the Internet by citing personal, academic, or work-related needs. Therefore, we must be aware of the warning signs of internet addiction, and educate children, parents, friends, and family about the risks associated with excessive Internet use. Ultimately, it is never too late to help a person who may be submerged and trapped in the complexity of the network.

For information on Internet addiction and other mental health issues, contact the National Institute of Mental Health at 1-866-615-NIMH (6464) (toll-free for those living in the United States) or visit their website at http://www.nimh.nih.gov. You can also reach them via email at nimhinfo@nih.gov.

Bibliography

Ankuta, George Y. y Abeles, Norman (1993). "Client Satisfaction, Clinical Significance and Meaningful Changes in Psychotherapy". Professional Psychology; Research and Practice, Vol. 24. No.1, 70-74. American Psychological Association, Inc.

https://www.ctg.albany.edu/media/pubs/pdfs/field_test.pdf

Kaplan And Sadock's Synopsis of Psychiatry by Benjamin J Sadock 11th edition (2014).

Cerniglia L, Zoratto F, Cimino S, Laviola G, Ammaniti M, Adriani W. Internet Addiction in adolescence: Neurobiological, psychosocial and clinical issues. Neurosci Biobehav Rev. 2017 May;76(Pt A):174-184. doi: 10.1016/j. neubiorev.2016.12.024. Epub 2016 Dec 24. PMID: 28027952.

Dean, W., Talbot, S., & Dean, A. (2019). Reframing Clinician Distress: Moral Injury Not Burnout. Federal practitioner: for the health care professionals of the VA, DoD, and PHS, 36(9), 400–402.

RISK FACTORS FOR INJURY TO WOMEN FROM DOMESTIC VIOLENCE DE- METRIOS N. KYRIACOU,

M.D., PH.D., DEIRDRE ANGLIN, M.D., M.P.H., ELLEN TALIAFERRO, M.D., SUSAN STONE, M.D., M.P.H., TONI TUBB, M.D., JUDITH A. LINDEN, M.D., ROBERT MUELLEMAN, M.D., ERIK BARTON, M.D., AND JESS F. KRAUS, PH.D., M.P.H. December 16, 1999 N Engl J Med 1999; 341:1892-1898.

Di chiara, 2000.

Echeburúa, Enrique & Gargallo, Paz. (2010). Adicción a las nuevas tecnologías y a las redes sociales en jóvenes: un nuevo reto. Adicciones: Revista de socidrogalcohol, ISSN 0214-4840, Vol. 22, N°. 2, 2010, pp. 91-96. 22. 10.20882/adicciones.196.

Emergencias psiquiátricas, Dr. Bartoli.

Farberowy Gordon in 1981. (John D. Weaver, Disasters: mental health interventions, pp. 7 y 31).

Frezza Md E. Moral Injury: The Pandemic for Physicians. Tex Med. 2019 Mar 1;115(3):4-6. PMID: 32084289.

Gálvez-Sánchez, C. M., Duschek, S., & Reyes Del Paso, G. A. (2019). Psycho- logical impact of fibromyalgia: current perspectives. Psychology research and behavior management, 12, 117–127. Retrieved from https://doi. org/10.2147/ PRBM.S178240

Hazlett SB, McCarthy ML, Londner MS, Onylke CU. Epidemiology of adult psychiatric visits to US emergency departments. Acad Emerg Med. 2004 Feb;11(2):193-5. PMID: 14759965.

Inanici F, Yunus MB. History of fibromyalgia: past to present. Curr Pain Headache Rep. 2004 Oct;8(5):369-78. doi: 10.1007/s11916-996-0010-6. PMID: 15361321.

Psychiatry, Janis L. Cutler. (2010).

Journal of Clinical Psychiatry. (2006).

Krishnamurthy S, Chetlapalli SK. Internet addiction: Prevalence and risk factors: A cross-sectional study among college students in Bengaluru, the Silicon Valley of India. Indian J Public Health. 2015 Apr-Jun;59(2):115-21. doi: 10.4103/0019-557X.157531. PMID: 26021648.

Lai J, Ma S, Wang Y, Cai Z, Hu J, Wei N, Wu J, Du H, Chen T, Li R, Tan H, Kang L, Yao L, Huang M, Wang H, Wang G, Liu Z, Hu S. Factors Associated With Mental Health Outcomes Among Health Care Workers Exposed to Coronavirus Disease 2019. JAMA Netw Open. 2020 Mar 2;3(3):e203976. doi: 10.1001/jamanetworkopen.2020.3976. PMID: 32202646; PMCID: PMC7090843.

Lee BH, Lee HK. Longitudinal study shows that addictive Internet use du- ring adolescence was associated with heavy drinking and smoking cigarettes in early adulthood. Acta Paediatr. 2017 Mar;106(3):497-502. doi: 10.1111/ apa.13706. Epub 2017 Jan 11. PMID: 27977879.

Lee, J. H., Mayeux, R., Mayo, D., Mo, J., Santana, V., Williamson, J., Flaquer, A., Ciappa, A., Rondon, H., Estevez, P., Lantigua, R., Kawarai, T., Toulina, A., Medrano, M., Torres, M., Stern, Y., Tycko, B., Rogaeva, E., St George-Hyslop, P., & Knowles, J. A. (2004). Fine mapping of 10q and 18q for familial Alzheimer's disease in Caribbean Hispanics. Molecular psychiatry, 9(11), 1042–1051. https:// doi.org/10.1038/sj.mp.4001538

Levenson, psychosomatic medicine. (2007).

avrogiorgou, P., Brüne, M., & Juckel, G. (2011). The management of psychiatric emergencies. Deutsches Arzteblatt International, 108(13), 222–230. https://doi. org/10.3238/arztebl.2011.0222.

https://www.mayoclinic.org/diseases-conditions/fibromyalgia/ symptoms-causes/syc-20354780

Munno D, Cappellin F, Saroldi M, Bechon E, Guglielmucci F, Passera R, Zullo G. Internet Addiction Disorder: Personality characteristics and risk of pathological overuse in adolescents. Psychiatry Res. 2017 Feb;248:1-5. doi: 10.1016/j.psychres.2016.11.008. Epub 2016 Nov 10. PMID: 27988425.

Muñoz, Manuel & Pérez Santos, Eloisa & Crespo, Maria & Guillén, Ana. (2009). Estigma y enfermedad mental. Análisis del rechazo social que sufren las personas con enfermedad mental.

Nakayama H, Mihara S, Higuchi S. Treatment and risk factors of Internet use disorders. Psychiatry Clin Neurosci. 2017 July;71(7):492-505. doi: 10.1111/ pcn.12493. Epub 2017 Feb 10. PMID: 27987253.

National Center for Statistics and Analysis. (2015). http://www. nimh.nih.gov.

Pedrelli, P., Shapero, B., Archibald, A., & Dale, C. (2016). Alcohol use and depression during adolescence and young adulthood: a summary and interpretation of mixed findings. Current addiction reports, 3(1), 91–97. https:// doi.org/10.1007/s40429-016-0084-0

Peele S. The Pleasure Principle in Addiction. Journal of Drug Issues. 1985;15(2):193-201. doi:10.1177/002204268501500203

http://www.postpartum.net

https://www.ptsd.va.gov/about/divisions/executive/norman_s. asp

Ripp, J., Peccoralo, L., & Charney, D. (2020). Attending to the Emotional Well-Being of the Health Care Workforce in a New York City Health System During the COVID-19 Pandemic. Academic medicine: journal of the Association of American Medical Colleges, 95(8), 1136–1139. https://doi.org/10.1097/ ACM.0000000000003414

R Russell IJ, Orr MD, Littman B, Vipraio GA, Alboukrek D, Michalek JE, Lopez Y, MacKillip F. Elevated cerebrospinal fluid levels of substance P in patients with the fibromyalgia syndrome. Arthritis Rheum. 1994 Nov;3 7(11):1593-601. doi: 10.1002/art.1780371106. PMID: 7526868.ussell IJ, Orr MD, Littman B, Vipraio GA, Alboukrek D, Michalek JE, Lopez Y, MacKillip F. Elevated cerebros- pinal fluid levels of substance P in patients with the fibromyalgia syndrome. Arthritis Rheum. 1994 Nov;37(11):1593-601. doi: 10.1002/art.1780371106. PMID: 7526868.

Sarris, J., O'Neil, A., Coulson, C.E. et al. Lifestyle medicine for depression. BMC Psychiatry 14, 107 (2014). https://doi.org/10.1186/1471-244X-14-107

http://www.sbpep.org

Song J, Park JH, Han DH, Roh S, Son JH, Choi TY, Lee H, Kim TH, Lee YS. Comparative study of the effects of bupropion and escitalopram on Internet gaming disorder. Psychiatry Clin Neurosci. 2016 Nov;70(11):527-535. doi: 10.1111/pcn.12429. Epub 2016 Oct 27. PMID: 27487975.

Sudarsanan, S., Chaudhury, S., Pawar, A. A., Salujha, S. K., & Srivastava, K. (2004). Psychiatric Emergencies. Medical journal, Armed Forces India, 60(1), 59–62. https://doi.org/10.1016/S0377-1237(04)80162-X

Weng, Chuan-Bu. (2013).

Widyanto L, McMurran M. The psychometric properties of the internet addiction test. Cyberpsychol Behav. 2004

Aug;7(4):443-50. doi: 10.1089/ cpb.2004.7.443. PMID: 15331031.

White et al, 1999 ARTHRITIS & RHEUMATISM Vol. 42, No. 1, January 1999, pp 76–83 © 1999, American College of Rheumatology.

Yuan, K., Qin, W., Wang, G., Zeng, F., Zhao, L., Yang, X., Liu, P., Liu, J., Sun, J., von Deneen, K. M., Gong, Q., Liu, Y., & Tian, J. (2011). Microstructure abnormalities in adolescents with internet addiction disorder. PloS one, 6(6), e20708. https://doi.org/10.1371/journal.pone.0020708.

About the author

Dr. Hernández was born in 1973 in Ensanche Julia, Santiago, Dominican Republic. He showed an interest in helping others from a young age and was elected vice president of the Rotaract Club of Santiago Apóstol La Esperanza of Rotary International during his high school years. In 1990, he received a Medal of Honor and a bachelor's degree in physical sciences and mathematics from Liceo Ulises Francisco Espaillat.

He graduated with a medical degree from Pontificia Universidad Católica Madre y Maestra (PUCMM) in 1996 and went on to become an assistant professor at the PUCMM School of Medicine from 1996 to 1998. In 1998, he was selected as one of the ten most talented young people in Santiago by the Presidency of the Dominican Republic.

Dr. Hernández is a member of various organizations, associations, and professional societies, including the American Medical Association (AMA), the American Psychiatric Association (APA), the Dominican Medical Association (DMA), Inc. of New York, the Dominican American National Roundtable (DNAR), Rosicrucian Order (AMORC), and the lodges of New York City, Fraternity 387 and Juan Pablo Duarte.

He was elected president of the Dominican Medical Association (DMA) in 2007-08 and re-elected in 2009-10. Currently, he serves as the president of the DMA board of directors. Over the past eighteen years, he has transformed the DMA with his hard work and visionary ideas, making him one of the most influential and powerful voices of the organization.

As a psychiatrist, Dr. Hernández continues to serve the Dominican community. He has gained prestige for his leadership in the Hispanic community, recognized by Telemundo International's "Día a Día" television program in 2007, "Herencia Hispana" by the Bronx Dominican Stop, and "the Dominican Gold Shield" in 2011. He has published many articles of interest to the local and international community.

Dr. Hernández has received numerous citations, recognitions, and awards, including citations from assemblymen, councilmen, and Dominican congressmen in Manhattan, the 2018 Illustrious Latino Awards, Instituto Duartiano, and Medicoop. He is also featured in the book "100 líderes dominicanos en Nueva York" published in 2011.

Dr. Hernández has a private psychiatric practice, Global Psychiatric Services (GPS), in Manhattan Borough, New York City, which he has run for almost a decade. In his free time, he enjoys playing chess, painting, writing poetry, and exploring mysticism. An annual chess tournament held in New York bears his name since 2015. He has also dabbled in acting and executive producing seven short films and movies, as well as community theater. Some of his poems have been transformed into songs.

Dr. Hernández is the father of two sons, Elmer Akhenaton and Armani Enoch, who are his inspiration. He is married to Olga Bourdierd, his support and blessing. His beloved mother Juana Hernández, his dear sister Rafaelina Hernández, and his late father are his motivation, giving him the strength and love to serve others.

An honest witness tells the truth,
but a false witness tells lies.
The words of the reckless pierce like swords,
but the tongue of the wise brings healing.
Truthful lips endure forever,
but a lying tongue lasts only a moment.
Deceit is in the hearts of those who plot evil,
but those who promote peace have joy.
(New International Version, 2011, Proverbs 12:17-20)

Do not repay anyone evil for evil.
Be careful to do what is right in the eyes of everyone.
On the contrary: "If your enemy is hungry, feed him;
if he is thirsty, give him something to drink.
In doing this, you will heap burning coals on his head."
Do not be overcome by evil, but overcome evil with good.
(New International Version, 2011, Romans 12:17, 20-21)

www.ingramcontent.com/pod-product-compliance
Lightning Source LLC
Chambersburg PA
CBHW051430150726
48000CB00005B/2027